Patients, Doctors, and Illness

# THE SOCIAL MEDICINE READER

**Second edition**

**VOLUME I** Patients, Doctors, and Illness

NANCY M. P. KING

RONALD P. STRAUSS

LARRY R. CHURCHILL

SUE E. ESTROFF

GAIL E. HENDERSON

JONATHAN OBERLANDER

*editors*

DUKE UNIVERSITY PRESS

*Durham and London 2005*

© 2005 Duke University Press • All rights reserved
Printed in the United States of America on acid-free paper ∞
Typeset in Trump Mediaeval by Keystone Typesetting, Inc.
Library of Congress Cataloging-in-Publication Data
appear on the last printed page of this book.
2nd printing, 2007

# Contents

## Preface to the Second Edition

Of the six editors of this second edition of the *Social Medicine Reader*, five are current members and one a former member of the Department of Social Medicine, University of North Carolina at Chapel Hill School of Medicine. Founded in 1977, the Department of Social Medicine includes scholars in medicine, the social sciences, the humanities, and public health. Its mission is to inform the work and thought of researchers, teachers, and practitioners on the social conditions and characteristics of patients, causes of illness, and barriers to effective care; and the responsibilities of the medical profession and other medical institutions.

This reader is based on the syllabus of a year-long, required, interdisciplinary course, Medicine and Society, which has been taught to first-year students at the University of North Carolina at Chapel Hill School of Medicine since 1978. The goal of the course since its inception has been to demonstrate that medicine and medical practice have a profound influence on—and are influenced by—social, cultural, political, and economic forces. Teaching this perspective requires integrating medical and nonmedical materials and viewpoints. This reader, therefore, arises not from one or two academic disciplines, but from many fields within medicine, the social sciences, and humanities.

With health care and health so central to the political, personal, and financial discourse of the day, this reader provides a starting point for informed, critical analysis. The three volumes of the *Social Medicine Reader* represent the most engaging, provocative, and informative materials and issues we have traversed with our students. While the origin of these volumes lies in the teaching of medical students, the selections were deliberately made with an eye toward engaging nonmedical readers, both from the interested public and from students in the arts and sciences.

The selections challenge standard ways of thinking about medical categories of disease, social categories of risk, and the types of moral reasoning on which much of the field of bioethics has been based. Their many voices include individual narratives of illness experience, commentaries by physicians, debate about complex medical cases, and conceptually and empirically based writings by scholars in medicine, the social sciences, and humanities. These are readings with the literary and scholarly power to convey the complicated relationships between medicine, health, and society. They do not resolve the most vexing contemporary issues but illuminate them.

Medicine's impact on society is multidimensional. Biomedical technology and practice, including its latest expression, genomic medicine, have profoundly affected our institutions and our social relations. Medicine has affected how we think about the most fundamental, enduring human experiences—conception, birth, maturation, sickness, suffering, healing, aging, and death—and it has shaped the metaphors we use to express our deepest concerns. Medical practices and our responses to them have helped to redefine the meaning of age, race, and gender. Technological advances in medicine have produced ethical dilemmas expressed in new vocabularies of science and economics, as well as in the familiar languages of morality and human relationships.

Social influences on medicine are apparent in several ways. First, modern science presumes that the pursuit of knowledge can and should be conducted with an unwavering adherence to neutral, objective observation and experimentation. Yet medical knowledge and practice, like all knowledge and practice, is shaped by political, cultural, and economic forces, within which doctors' ideas about disease—in fact their very definitions of disease—depend on the roles science and scientists play in particular cultures, as well as on the cultures of laboratory and clinical science. Medicine tends to reduce the world to a vocabulary of its own, one that seems immune to the vagaries and vicissitudes of culture. But diseases are not immutable; they are shaped by person, time, and place, and are identified and endowed with significance only within social and cultural contexts.

Despite the power of the biomedical model of disease and the increasing specificity of molecular and genetic knowledge, social factors have always influenced the occurrence and course of most diseases. And once disease has occurred, the power of medicine to alter its course is constrained by the larger social and economic context. Beyond these problems, many medical interventions are themselves of contested or unclear value. Spending on health care in the United States has long outstripped that of other industrialized nations, but that spending has not resulted in a healthier population. What does our medicine produce? Who benefits from these enormous expenditures of resources?

Repeatedly, the readings throughout these three volumes make clear that much of what we encounter in science, in society, and in everyday and extraordinary lives is indeterminate, ambiguous, complex, and contradictory. And because of this inherent ambiguity, the interwoven selections highlight conflicts—conflict about power and authority, autonomy and choice, security and risk. By critically analyzing these and many other related issues, we can open up possibilities, change what seems inevitable, and practice medical education and doctoring with an increased capacity for reflection and self-examination. The goal is to ignite and to fuel the inner voices of social, human, and moral analysis among health care professionals, and among us all.

Any collection of readings like the three volumes that make up the *Social Medicine Reader* is open to challenges about what has been included and what has been left out. This collection is no exception. The study of medicine and society is dynamic, with large and ever expanding bodies of new literature from which to draw. We have omitted some readings widely considered "classics" and included some readings that are classic only in our experience. We have chosen to include material with literary and scholarly merit and that has worked well in the classroom, provoking discussion and engaging readers' imaginations. These readings invite self-conscious, multilevel, critical examination, a work of reading and discussion that is inherently difficult but educationally rewarding.

The first edition of the *Social Medicine Reader* was a single volume. We decided to make the second edition three volumes to facilitate use by different audiences with different interests; however, the three volumes also function as an integrated whole. Volume I, *Patients, Doctors, and Illness*, examines the experience of illness, the roles and training of health care professionals and their relationships with patients, ethics in health care, and experiences and decisions at the end of life. It includes fiction and nonfiction narratives and poetry; definitions and case-based discussions of moral precepts in health care, such as truth telling, informed consent, privacy, autonomy, and beneficence; and scholarly readings providing legal, ethical, and practical perspectives on many familiar but persistent ethical and social questions raised by illness and health care. Volume II, *Social and Cultural Contributions to Health, Difference, and Inequality,* explores health and illness, focusing on how difference and disability are defined and experienced in contemporary America and how the social categories commonly used to predict disease outcomes—gender, race/ethnicity, and social class—have become contested terrain. Narratives and essays feature individuals managing illness in daily life, and families both coping with and contributing to the challenges of ill health. Social epidemiological categories are examined empirically and critically. Volume III, *Health Policy, Markets, and Medicine*, examines issues and controversies in health policy. Essays analyze a broad spectrum of topics, from the historical forces that shaped development of the American health system to contemporary reform debates over controlling medical care spending and covering the uninsured. International health systems, medical care rationing, and emerging policy issues—including the rise of consumer-driven insurance and population aging—are also explored.

We thank our teaching colleagues who helped create and refine both the first and the second editions of this reader. These colleagues have come over the years from both within and outside the Department of Social Medicine and the University of North Carolina at Chapel Hill. Equal gratitude goes to our students, whose criticism and enthusiasm over two decades have improved our teaching and have influenced us greatly in making the selections for the reader. The leadership of Department of Social Medicine chairs and course directors since 1978 has also been invaluable. We thank the department's faculty and staff, past and present; we especially thank Judy Benoit, for many years the Medicine and Society course coordinator, and Jeff Kim, our student research assistant. In addition, Larry Churchill thanks the faculty who have taught with him in the Ecology of Health Care course at Vanderbilt School of Medicine during 2002 and 2003 for their many ideas for improving the second edition of the reader. Jon Oberlander gratefully acknowledges the support of the Greenwall Foundation and its Faculty Scholars Program in Bioethics. The editors gratefully acknowledge support from the Department of Social Medicine, University of North Carolina at Chapel Hill School of Medicine, and the Center for Clinical and Research Ethics, Vanderbilt University.

**Patients, Doctors, and Illness**

# Introduction

This first volume in a series of three that comprise the *Social Medicine Reader* thematically explores the experience of illness; the roles and training of health care professionals and their relationships with patients; ethics in health care; and experiences and decisions at the end of life. The volume's readings, which include narratives, essays, case studies, fiction, and poetry, have been "road-tested" in social science, ethics, and humanities classes in health professional schools and graduate and undergraduate programs. We cannot and do not cover any content area completely; our goal instead is to provide stimulating selected readings from which to launch discussion and debate.

The six editors of this volume are diverse in scholarly backgrounds, knowledge and expertise, and teaching styles. We each teach the same materials differently, but have learned much from each other through many years of faculty meetings. Our collaboration exemplifies the adaptability of the volume's readings to a variety of formats, settings, and approaches.

The readings have been used as triggers for debate, small group interactions or exercises, and launching points for discussions, at many levels and in many directions. Even teachers and students unaccustomed to considering fiction and poetry may be surprised at how readily these materials can stimulate rich and nuanced discussion of profoundly significant issues—especially when read aloud.

Beginning this volume with the experience of illness helps to ground the nature and meaning of sickness and healing in the familiar but unique experience of being a patient. All health care providers have been, and will be again, patients and the family members of patients. Vivid narratives of managing illness in daily life help build understanding of the vantage point of the patient and of family members who participate in the illness experience. Much illness is cared for in the family context; families guide health choices, provide healing, and interact with the health system, helping to negotiate its challenges and complexities. Patients and families grieve and laugh together, trust their doctors, and challenge them.

In the second part of the volume, medical socialization and the doctor-patient relationship are considered. Social scientists have extensively examined the social processes that transform medical students into counselors and interveners in issues of life and death. Professions, like other social groups, have cultures: they have specialized languages and ways of understanding, norms of behavior, unique customs, rites of passage, and codes of conduct. The "culture of medicine" is transmitted in a training process that changes the student through direct contact with and knowledge of the most private aspects of human existence. Many students enter medical school with idealistic views of medicine and its goals. As they learn the ideology and ethics of medicine, they may face dilemmas that are rarely voiced in public; they may undergo profound changes in their perspectives and even their identities. These readings promote reflection upon the roles of health professional students and practitioners, on the challenges inherent in the physician-patient relationship, and on navigating between professional and personal experiences and values.

The third part of the volume continues the progression of themes by enlarging discussion to include health care ethics and the roles of professionals. Readings examine moral reasoning and what it means to have a moral life as a health care professional in relationships with patients. Fundamental moral precepts in health care practice—truth telling, informed consent, privacy, autonomy, and beneficence—are presented in cases and stories that pose problems to be unraveled, examined, and debated from a wide range of viewpoints. Each quandary is presented not as a syllogism but as a dynamic experience: issues embedded in time, place, society, history, and culture, and entangled in multiple relationships. The scholarly literature addressing ethics in medicine is voluminous and is in no way recapitulated in this section; instead, we expect readers to find their own ways, through reading and discussion, to insights that can parallel those of the best thinkers, but that mean more for being discovered rather than decreed.

The final part of this volume employs the prior themes to address end-of-life decision making. The work of this section includes an effort to clarify concepts; an examination of disagreements and decision-making dilemmas through moral argument and appreciation of the personal, professional, social, and emotional contexts of these decisions; and specific attention to life prolongation, treatment withdrawal, and the ending of life, whether deliberate or unwelcome. Many questions are raised about the legal, ethical, and practical medical aspects of end-of-life care, the nature and power of medical judgments, and long-standing professional and personal disagreements about the end of life that have yet to be resolved. A selection of remarkably vivid poetry opens the possibility for discussion of mortality, meaning, loss, and grief. Once again, we have chosen only a few selections from voluminous and growing literatures in such fields as advance care planning and assisted suicide, and such diverse materials as legal statutes and cases, empirical studies, and narratives both fictional and documentary in nature. Yet we are confident that the selection we have made is rich and deep enough to sustain critical reflection and thoughtful discussion.

The variety of readings in this volume can be addressed productively from many disciplinary perspectives and many teaching styles and formats. They can be reshuffled and recombined, stand together or alone, or be supplemented by other literature. The key requirement for using these readings successfully is to approach them with flexibility—not as containing the right answers but as helping to shape the right questions. If our experience as teachers is any guide, both teachers and students of materials like these will go on asking the questions, and finding different and deeper answers, all their lives.

# PART I

**The Experience of Illness**

# The Nature of Suffering and the Goals of Medicine
Eric J. Cassell

The obligation of physicians to relieve human suffering stretches back into antiquity. Despite this fact, little attention is explicitly given to the problem of suffering in medical education, research, or practice. I will begin by focusing on a modern paradox: Even in the best settings and with the best physicians, it is not uncommon for suffering to occur not only during the course of a disease but also as a result of its treatment. To understand this paradox and its resolution requires an understanding of what suffering is and how it relates to medical care.

Consider this case: A 35-year-old sculptor with metastatic disease of the breast was treated by competent physicians employing advanced knowledge and technology and acting out of kindness and true concern. At every stage, the treatment as well as the disease was a source of suffering to her. She was uncertain and frightened about her future, but she could get little information from her physicians, and what she was told was not always the truth. She had been unaware, for example, that the irradiated breast would be so disfigured. After an oophorectomy and a regimen of medications, she became hirsute, obese, and devoid of libido. With tumor in the supraclavicular fossa, she lost strength in the hand that she had used in sculpturing, and she became profoundly depressed. She had a pathologic fracture of the femur, and treatment was delayed while her physicians openly disagreed about pinning her hip.

Each time her disease responded to therapy and her hope was rekindled, a new manifestation would appear. Thus, when a new course of chemotherapy was started, she was torn between a desire to live and the fear that

Eric J. Cassell, "The Nature of Suffering and the Goals of Medicine," from *New England Journal of Medicine*, vol. 306, 639–645. © 1982 by the Massachusetts Medical Society. Reprinted by permission of the publisher.

allowing hope to emerge again would merely expose her to misery if the treatment failed. The nausea and vomiting from the chemotherapy were distressing, but no more so than the anticipation of hair loss. She feared the future. Each tomorrow was seen as heralding increased sickness, pain, or disability, never as the beginning of better times. She felt isolated because she was no longer like other people and could not do what other people did. She feared that her friends would stop visiting her. She was sure that she would die.

This young woman had severe pain and other physical symptoms that caused her suffering. But she also suffered from some threats that were social and from others that were personal and private. She suffered from the effects of the disease and its treatment on her appearance and abilities. She also suffered unremittingly from her perception of the future.

What can this case tell us about the ends of medicine and the relief of suffering? Three facts stand out: The first is that this woman's suffering was not confined to her physical symptoms. The second is that she suffered not only from her disease but also from its treatment. The third is that one could not anticipate what she would describe as a source of suffering; like other patients, she had to be asked. Some features of her condition she would call painful, upsetting, uncomfortable, and distressing, but not a source of suffering. In these characteristics her case was ordinary.

In discussing the matter of suffering with lay persons, I learned that they were shocked to discover that the problem of suffering was not directly addressed in medical education. My colleagues of a contemplative nature were surprised at how little they knew of the problem and how little thought they had given it, whereas medical students tended to be unsure of the relevance of the issue to their work.

The relief of suffering, it would appear, is considered one of the primary ends of medicine by patients and lay persons, but not by the medical profession. As in the case of the dying, patients and their friends and families do not make a distinction between physical and nonphysical sources of suffering in the same way that doctors do.[1]

A search of the medical and social-science literature did not help me in understanding what suffering is; the word "suffering" was most often coupled with the word "pain," as in "pain and suffering." (The data bases used were *Psychological Abstracts*, the *Citation Index*, and the *Index Medicus*.)

This phenomenon reflects a historically constrained and currently inadequate view of the ends of medicine. Medicine's traditional concern primarily for the body and for physical disease is well known, as are the widespread effects of the mind-body dichotomy on medical theory and practice. I believe that this dichotomy itself is a source of the paradoxical situation in which doctors cause suffering in their care of the sick. Today, as ideas about the separation of mind and body are called into question, physicians are concerning themselves with new aspects of the human condition. The profession of medicine is being pushed and pulled into new areas, both by its technology and by the demands of its patients. Attempting to understand what suffering is and how physicians might truly be devoted to its relief will require that medicine and its critics overcome the dichotomy between mind and body and the associated dichotomies between subjective and objective and between person and object.

In the remainder of this essay I am going to make three points. The first is that suffering is experienced by persons. In the separation between mind and body, the concept of the person, or personhood, has been associated with that of mind, spirit, and the subjective. However, as I will show, a person is not merely mind, merely spiritual, or only subjectively knowable. Personhood has many facets, and it is ignorance of them that actively contributes to patients' suffering. The understanding of the place of the person in human illness requires a rejection of the historical dualism of mind and body.

The second point derives from my interpretation of clinical observations: Suffering occurs when an impending destruction of the person is perceived; it continues until the threat of disintegration has passed or until the integrity of the person can be restored in some other manner. It follows, then, that although suffering often occurs in the presence of acute pain, shortness of breath, or other bodily symptoms, suffering extends beyond the physical. Most generally, suffering can be defined as the state of severe distress associated with events that threaten the intactness of the person.

The third point is that suffering can occur in relation to any aspect of the person, whether it is in the realm of social roles, group identification, the relation with self, body, or family, or the relation with a transpersonal, transcendent source of meaning. Below is a simplified description or "topology" of the constituents of personhood.


### "Person" Is Not "Mind"

The split between mind and body that has so deeply influenced our approach to medical care was proposed by Descartes to resolve certain philosophical issues. Moreover, Cartesian dualism made it possible for science to escape the control of the church by assigning the noncorporeal, spiritual realm to the church, leaving the physical world as the domain of science. In that religious age, "person," synonymous with "mind," was necessarily off limits to science.

Changes in the meaning of concepts like that of personhood occur with changes in society, while the word for the concept remains the same. This fact tends to obscure the depth of the transformations that have occurred between the 17th century and today. People simply *are* "persons" in this time, as in past times, and they have difficulty imagining that the term described something quite different in an earlier period when the concept was more constrained.

If the mind-body dichotomy results in assigning the body to medicine, and the person is not in that category, then the only remaining place for the person is in the category of mind. Where the mind is problematic (not identifiable in objective terms), its very reality diminishes for science, and so, too, does that of the person. Therefore, so long as the mind-body dichotomy is accepted, suffering is either subjective and thus not truly "real"—not within medicine's domain—or identified exclusively with bodily pain. Not only is such an identification misleading and distorting, for it depersonalizes the sick patient, but it is itself a source of suffering. It is not possible to treat sickness as something that happens solely to the body without thereby risking damage to the person. An anachronistic division of the human condition into what is medical (having to do with the body) and what is nonmedical (the remainder) has given medicine too narrow a notion of its calling. Because of this division, physicians may, in concentrating on the cure of bodily disease, do things that cause the patient as a person to suffer.

### An Impending Destruction of Person

Suffering is ultimately a personal matter. Patients sometimes report suffering when one does not expect it, or do not report suffering when one does expect it. Furthermore, a person can suffer enormously at the distress of another, especially a loved one.

In some theologies, suffering has been seen as bringing one closer to God. This "function" of suffering is at once its glorification and its relief. If, through great pain or deprivation, someone is brought closer to a cherished goal, that person may have no sense of having suffered but may instead feel enormous triumph. To an observer, however, only the deprivation may be apparent. This cautionary note is important because people are often said to have suffered greatly, in a religious context, when they are known only to have been injured, tortured, or in pain, not to have suffered.

Although pain and suffering are closely identified in the medical literature, they are phenomenologically distinct.[2] The difficulty of understanding pain and the problems of physicians in providing adequate relief of physical pain are well known.[3-5]

The greater the pain, the more it is believed to cause suffering. However, some pain, like that of childbirth, can be extremely severe and yet considered rewarding. The perceived meaning of pain influences the amount of medication that will be required to control it. For example, a patient reported that when she believed the pain in her leg was sciatica, she could control it with small doses of codeine, but when she discovered that it was due to the spread of malignant disease, much greater amounts of medication were required for relief. Patients can writhe in pain from kidney stones and by their own admission not be suffering, because they "know what it is"; they may also report considerable suffering from apparently minor discomfort when they do not know its source. Suffering in close relation to the intensity of pain is reported when the pain is virtually overwhelming, such as that associated with a dissecting aortic aneurysm. Suffering is also reported when the patient does not believe that the pain can be controlled. The suffering of patients with terminal cancer can often be relieved by demonstrating that their pain truly can be controlled; they will then often tolerate the same pain without any medication, preferring the pain to the side effects of their analgesics. Another type of pain that can be a source of suffering is pain that is not overwhelming but continues for a very long time.

In summary, people in pain frequently report suffering from the pain when they feel out of control, when the pain is overwhelming, when the source of the pain is unknown, when the meaning of the pain is dire, or when the pain is chronic.

In all these situations, persons perceive pain as a threat to their continued existence—not merely to their lives, but to their integrity as persons. That this is the relation of pain to suffering is strongly suggested by the fact that suffering can be relieved, in the presence of continued pain, by making the source of the pain known, changing its meaning, and demonstrating that it can be controlled and that an end is in sight.

It follows, then, that suffering has a temporal element. In order for a situation to be a source of suffering, it must influence the person's perception of future events. ("If the pain continues like this, I *will be* overwhelmed"; "If the pain comes from cancer, I *will* die"; "If the pain cannot be controlled, I *will not* be able to take it.") At the moment when the patient is saying, "If the pain continues like this, I will be overwhelmed," he or she is not overwhelmed. Fear itself always involves the future. In the case with which I opened this essay, the patient could not give up her fears of her sense of future, despite the agony they caused her. As suffering is discussed in the other dimensions of personhood, note how it would not exist if the future were not a major concern.

Two other aspects of the relation between pain and suffering should be mentioned. Suffering can occur when physicians do not validate the patient's pain. In the absence of disease, physicians may suggest that the pain is "psychological" (in the sense of not being real) or that the patient is "faking." Similarly, patients with chronic pain may believe after a time that they can no longer talk to others about their distress. In the former case the person is caused to distrust his or her perceptions of reality, and in both instances social isolation adds to the person's suffering.

Another aspect essential to an understanding of the suffering of sick persons is the relation of meaning to the way in which illness is experienced. The word "meaning" is used here in two senses. In the first, to mean is to signify, to imply. Pain in the chest may imply heart disease. We also say that we know what something means when we know how important it is. The importance of things is always personal and individual, even though meaning in this sense may be shared by others or by society as a whole. What something signifies and how important it is relative to the whole array of a person's concerns contribute to its personal meaning. "Belief" is another word for that aspect of meaning concerned with implications, and "value" concerns the degree of importance to a particular person.

The personal meaning of things does not consist exclusively of values and beliefs that are held intellectually; it includes other dimensions. For the same word, a person may simultaneously have a cognitive meaning, an affective or emotional meaning, a bodily meaning, and a transcendent or spiritual meaning. And there may be contradictions in the different levels of meaning. The nuances of personal meaning are complex, and when I speak of personal meanings I am implying this complexity in all its depth—known and unknown. Personal meaning is a fundamental dimension of personhood, and there can be no understanding of human illness or suffering without taking it into account.

### A Simplified Description of the Person

A simple topology of a person may be useful in understanding the relation between suffering and the goals of medicine. The features discussed below point the way to further study and to the possibility of specific action by individual physicians.

Persons have personality and character. Personality traits appear within the first few weeks of life and are remarkably durable over time. Some personalities handle some illnesses better than others. Individual persons vary in character as well. During the heyday of psychoanalysis in the 1950s, all behavior was attributed to unconscious determinants: No one was bad or good; they were merely sick or well. Fortunately, that simplistic view of human character is now out of favor. Some people do in fact have stronger characters and bear adversity better. Some are good and kind under the stress of terminal illness, whereas others become mean and offensive when even mildly ill.

A person has a past. The experiences gathered during one's life are a part of today as well as yesterday. Memory exists in the nostrils and the hands, not only in the mind. A fragrance drifts by, and a memory is evoked. My feet have not forgotten how to roller-skate, and my hands remember skills that I was hardly aware I had learned. When these past experiences involve sickness and medical care, they can influence present illness and medical care. They stimulate fear, confidence, physical symptoms, and anguish. It damages people to rob them of their past and deny their memories, or to mock their fears and worries. A person without a past is incomplete.

Life experiences—previous illness, experiences with doctors, hospitals, and medications, deformities and disabilities, pleasures and successes, miseries and failures—all form the nexus for illness. The personal meaning of the disease and its treatment arises from the past as well as the present. If cancer occurs in a patient with self-confidence from past achievements, it may give rise to optimism and a resurgence of strength. Even if it is fatal, the disease may not produce the destruction of the person but, rather, reaffirm his or her indomitability. The outcome would be different in a person for whom life had been a series of failures.

The intensity of ties to the family cannot be overemphasized; people frequently behave as though they were physical extensions of their parents. Events that might cause suffering in others may be borne without complaint by someone who believes that the disease is part of his or her family identity and hence inevitable. Even diseases for which no heritable basis is known may be borne easily by a person because others in the family have been similarly afflicted. Just as the person's past experiences give meaning to present events, so do the past experiences of his or her family. Those meanings are part of the person.

A person has a cultural background. Just as a person is part of a culture and a society, these elements are part of the person. Culture defines what is meant by masculinity or femininity, what attire is acceptable, attitudes toward the dying and sick, mating behavior, the height of chairs and steps, degrees of tolerance for odors and excreta, and how the aged and the disabled are treated. Cultural definitions have an enormous impact on the sick and can be a source of untold suffering. They influence the behavior of others toward the sick person and that of the sick toward themselves. Cultural norms and social rules regulate whether someone can be among others or will be isolated, whether the sick will be considered foul or acceptable, and whether they are to be pitied or censured.

Returning to the sculptor described earlier, we know why that young woman suffered. She was housebound and bedbound, her face was changed by steroids, she was masculinized by her treatment, one breast was scarred, and she had almost no hair. The degree of importance attached to these losses—that aspect of their personal meaning—is determined to a great degree by cultural priorities.

With this in mind, we can also realize how much someone devoid of physical pain, even devoid of "symptoms," may suffer. People suffer from what they have lost of themselves in relation to the world of objects, events, and relationships. We realize, too, that although medical care can reduce the impact of sickness, inattentive care can increase the disruption caused by illness.

A person has roles. I am a husband, a father, a physician, a teacher, a brother, an orphaned son, and an uncle. People are their roles, and each role has rules. Together, the rules that guide the performance of roles make up a complex set of entitlements and limitations of responsibility and privilege. By middle age, the roles may be so firmly set that disease can lead to the virtual destruction of a person by making the performance of his or her roles impossible. Whether the patient is a doctor who cannot doctor or a mother who cannot mother, he or she is diminished by the loss of function.

No person exists without others; there is no consciousness without a consciousness of others, no speaker without a hearer, and no act, object, or thought that does not somehow encompass others.[6] All behavior is or will be involved with others, even if only in memory or reverie. Take away others, remove sight or hearing, and the person is diminished. Everyone dreads becoming blind or deaf, but these are only the most obvious injuries to human interaction. There are many ways in which human beings can be cut off from others and then suffer the loss.

It is in relationships with others that the full range of human emotions finds expression. It is this dimension of the person that may be injured when illness disrupts the ability to express emotion. Furthermore, the extent and nature of a sick person's relationships influence the degree of suffering from a disease. There is a vast difference between going home to an empty apartment and going home to a network of friends and family after hospitalization. Illness may occur in one partner of a long and strongly bound marriage or in a union that is falling apart. Suffering from the loss of sexual function associated with some diseases will depend not only on the importance of sexual performance itself but also on its importance in the sick person's relationships.

A person is a political being. A person is in this sense equal to other persons, with rights and obligations and the ability to redress injury by others and the state. Sickness can interfere, producing the feeling of political powerlessness and lack of representation. Persons who are permanently handicapped may suffer from a feeling of exclusion from participation in the political realm.

Persons do things. They act, create, make, take apart, put together, wind, unwind, cause to be, and cause to vanish. They know themselves, and are known, by these acts. When illness restricts the range of activity of persons, they are not themselves.

Persons are often unaware of much that happens within them and why. Thus, there are things in the mind that cannot be brought to awareness by ordinary reflection. The structure of the unconscious is pictured quite differently by different scholars, but most students of human behavior accept the assertion that such an interior world exists. People can behave in ways that seem inexplicable and strange even to themselves, and the sense of powerlessness that the person may feel in the presence of such behavior can be a source of great distress.

Persons have regular behaviors. In health, we take for granted the details of our day-to-day behavior. Persons know themselves to be well as much by whether they behave as usual as by any other set of facts. Patients decide that they are ill because they cannot perform as usual, and they may suffer the loss of their routine. If they cannot do the things that they identify with the fact of their being, they are not whole.

Every person has a body. The relation with one's body may vary from identification with it to admiration, loathing, or constant fear. The body may even be perceived as a representation of a parent, so that when something happens to the person's body it is as though a parent were injured. Disease can so alter the relation that the body is no longer seen as a friend but, rather, as an untrustworthy enemy. This is intensified if the illness comes on without warning, and as illness persists, the person may feel increasingly vulnerable. Just as many people have an expanded sense of self as a result of changes in their bodies from exercise, the potential exists for a contraction of this sense through injury to the body.

Everyone has a secret life. Sometimes it takes the form of fantasies and dreams of glory; sometimes it has a real existence known to only a few. Within the secret life are fears, desires, love affairs of the past and present, hopes, and fantasies. Disease may destroy not only the public or the private person but the secret person as well. A secret beloved friend may be lost to a sick person because he or she has no legitimate place by the sickbed. When that happens, the patient may have lost the part of life that made tolerable an otherwise embittered existence. Or the loss may be only of a dream, but one that might have come true. Such loss can be a source of great distress and intensely private pain.

Everyone has a perceived future. Events that one expects to come to pass vary from expectations for one's children to a belief in one's creative ability. Intense unhappiness results from a loss of the future—the future of the individual person, of children, and of other loved ones. Hope dwells in this dimension of existence, and great suffering attends the loss of hope.

Everyone has a transcendent dimension, a life of the spirit. This is most directly expressed in religion and the mystic traditions, but the frequency with which people have intense feelings of bonding with groups, ideals, or anything larger and more enduring than the person is evidence of the universality of the transcendent dimension. The quality of being greater and more lasting than an individual life gives this aspect of the person its timeless dimension. The profession of medicine appears to ignore the human spirit. When I see patients in nursing homes who have become only bodies, I wonder whether it is not their transcendent dimension that they have lost.

### The Nature of Suffering

For purposes of explanation, I have outlined various parts that make up a person. However, persons cannot be reduced to their parts in order to be better understood. Reductionist scientific methods, so successful in human biology, do not help us to comprehend whole persons. My intent was rather to suggest the complexity of the person and the potential for injury and suffering that exists in everyone. With this in mind, any suggestion of mechanical simplicity should disappear from my definition of suffering. All the aspects of personhood—the lived past, the family's lived past, culture and society, roles, the instrumental dimension, associations and relationships, the body, the unconscious mind, the political being, the secret life, the perceived future, and the transcendent dimension—are susceptible to damage and loss.

Injuries to the integrity of the person may be expressed by sadness, anger, loneliness, depression, grief, unhappiness, melancholy, rage, withdrawal, or yearning. We acknowledge the person's right to have and express such feelings. But we often forget that the affect is merely the outward expression of the injury, not the injury itself. We know little about the nature of the injuries themselves, and what we know has been learned largely from literature, not medicine.

If the injury is sufficient, the person suffers. The only way to learn what damage is sufficient to cause suffering, or whether suffering is present, is to ask the sufferer. We all recognize certain injuries that almost invariably cause suffering: the death or distress of loved ones, powerlessness, helplessness, hopelessness, torture, the loss of a life's work, betrayal, physical agony, isolation, homelessness, memory failure, and fear. Each is both universal and individual. Each touches features common to all of us, yet each contains features that must be defined in terms of a specific person at a specific time. With the relief of suffering in mind, however, we should reflect on how remarkably little is known of these injuries.

### The Amelioration of Suffering

One might inquire why everyone is not suffering all the time. In a busy life, almost no day passes in which one's intactness goes unchallenged. Obviously, not every challenge is a threat. Yet I suspect that there is more suffering than is known. Just as people with chronic pain learn to keep it to themselves because others lose interest, so may those with chronic suffering.

There is another reason why every injury may not cause suffering. Persons are able to enlarge themselves in response to damage, so that instead of being reduced, they may indeed grow. This response to suffering has encouraged the belief that suffering is good for people. To some degree, and in some persons, this may be so. If a leg is injured so that an athlete cannot run again, the athlete may compensate for the loss by learning another sport or mode of expression. So it is with the loss of relationships, loves, roles, physical strength, dreams, and power. The human body may lack the capacity to gain a new part when one is lost, but the person has it.

The ability to recover from loss without succumbing to suffering is sometimes called resilience, as though nothing but elastic rebound were involved, but it is more as though an inner force were withdrawn from one manifestation of a person and redirected to another. If a child dies and the parent makes a successful recovery, the person is said to have "rebuilt" his or her life. The term suggests that the parts of the person are structured in a new manner, allowing expression in different dimensions. If a previously active person is confined to a wheelchair, intellectual pursuits may occupy more time.

Recovery from suffering often involves help, as though people who have lost parts of themselves can be sustained by the personhood of others until their own recovers. This is one of the latent functions of physicians: to lend strength. A group, too, may lend strength: Consider the success of groups of the similarly afflicted in easing the burden of illness (e.g., women with mastectomies, people with ostomies, and even the parents or family members of the diseased).

Meaning and transcendence offer two additional ways by which the suffering associated with destruction of a part of personhood is ameliorated. Assigning a meaning to the injurious condition often reduces or even resolves the suffering associated with it. Most often, a cause for the condition is sought within past behaviors or beliefs. Thus, the pain or threat that causes suffering is seen as not destroying a part of the person, because it is part of the person by virtue of its origin within the self. In our culture, taking the blame for harm that comes to oneself because of the unconscious mind serves the same purpose as the concept of karma in Eastern theologies; suffering is reduced when it can be located within a coherent set of meanings. Physicians are familiar with the question from the sick, "Did I do something that made this happen?" It is more tolerable for a terrible thing to happen because of something that one has done than it is to be at the mercy of chance.

Transcendence is probably the most powerful way in which one is restored to wholeness after an injury to personhood. When experienced, transcendence locates the person in a far larger landscape. The sufferer is not isolated by pain but is brought closer to a transpersonal source of meaning and to the human community that shares those meanings. Such an experience need not involve religion in any formal sense; however, in its transpersonal dimension, it is deeply spiritual. For example, patriotism can be a secular expression of transcendence.

### When Suffering Continues

But what happens when suffering is not relieved? If suffering occurs when there is a threat to one's integrity or a loss of a part of a person, then suffering will continue if the person cannot be made whole again. Little is known about this aspect of suffering. Is much of what we call depression merely unrelieved suffering? Considering that depression commonly follows the loss of loved ones, business reversals, prolonged illness, profound injuries to self-esteem, and other damages to personhood, the possibility is real. In many chronic or serious diseases, persons who "recover" or who seem to be successfully treated do not return to normal function. They may never again be employed, recover sexual function, pursue career goals, reestablish family relationships, or reenter the social world, despite a physical cure. Such patients may not have recovered from the nonphysical changes occurring with serious illness. Consider the dimensions of personhood described above, and note that each is threatened or damaged in profound illness. It should come as no surprise, then, that chronic suffering frequently follows in the wake of disease.

The paradox with which this essay began—that suffering is often caused by the treatment of the sick—no longer seems so puzzling. How could it be otherwise, when medicine has concerned itself so little with the nature and causes of suffering? This lack is not a failure of good intentions. None are more concerned about pain or loss of function than physicians. Instead, it is a failure of knowledge and understanding. We lack knowledge, because in working from a dichotomy contrived within a historical context far from our own, we have artificially circumscribed our task in caring for the sick.

Attempts to understand all the known dimensions of personhood and their relations to illness and suffering present problems of staggering complexity. The problems are no greater, however, than those initially posed by the question of how the body works—a question that we have managed to answer in extraordinary detail. If the ends of medicine are to be directed toward the relief of human suffering, the need is clear.

## Notes

I am indebted to Rabbi Jack Bemporad; to Drs. Joan Cassell, Peter Dineen, Nancy McKenzie, and Richard Zaner; to Ms. Dawn McGuire; to the members of the Research Group on Death, Suffering, and Well-Being of The Hastings Center for their advice and assistance; and to the Arthur Vining Davis Foundations for support of the research group.

1   Cassell, E. Being and becoming dead. Soc Res. 1972; 39:528–42.
2   Bakan, D. Disease, pain and sacrifice: toward a psychology of suffering. Chicago: Beacon Press, 1971.
3   Marks, R.M., Sachar, E.J. Undertreatment of medical inpatients with narcotic analgesics. Ann Intern Med. 1973; 78:173–81.
4   Kanner, R.M., Foley, K.M. Patterns of narcotic drug use in a cancer pain clinic. Ann NY Acad Sci. 1981; 362:161–72.
5   Goodwin, J.S., Goodwin, J.M., Vogel, A.V. Knowledge and use of placebos by house officers and nurses. Ann Intern Med. 1979; 91:106–10.
6   Zaner, R. The context of self: a phenomenological inquiry using medicine as a clue. Athens: Ohio University Press, 1981.

## Lilacs in September
Katha Pollitt

Shocked to the root
like the lilac bush
in the vacant lot
by the hurricane—

whose black branch split
by wind or rain
has broken out
unseasonably

into these scant ash-
colored blossoms
lifted high
as if to say

to passersby
*What will unleash
itself in you
when your storm comes?*

Katha Pollitt, "Lilacs in September," from *The New Yorker*, 22 September 2003, 189. © 2003 by Condé Nast Publications. Reprinted by permission of the publisher.

# Diabetes
James Dickey

I

*Sugar*

One night I thirsted like a prince
Then like a king
Then like an empire    like a world
On fire. I rose and flowed away and fell
Once more to sleep. In an hour I was back
In the kingdom    staggering, my belly going round with self-
Made night-water, wondering what
The hell. Months of having a tongue
Of flame convinced me: I had better not go
On this way. The doctor was young

And nice. He said, I must tell you,
My friend, that it is needles moderation
And exercise. You don't want to look forward
To gangrene and kidney

Failure    boils blindness infection skin trouble falling
Teeth coma and death.
O.K.
In sleep my mouth went dry
With my answer    and in it burned the sands
Of time with new fury. Sleep could give me no water
But my own. Gangrene in white

James Dickey, "Diabetes," from *The Eye-Beaters, Blood, Victory, Madness, Buckhead, and Mercy.* © 1969 by Doubleday. Reprinted by permission of Random House, Inc.

Was in my wife's hand at breakfast
Heaped like a mountain. Moderation, moderation,
My friend, and exercise. Each time the barbell
Rose    each time a foot fell
Jogging, it counted itself
One death    two death    three death and resurrection
For a little while. Not bad! I always knew it would have to be
somewhere around
The house: the real
Symbol of Time I could eat
And live with, coming true when I opened my mouth:
True in the coffee and the child's birthday
Cake    helping sickness be fire-
tongued, sleepless and water-
logged    but not bad, sweet sand
Of time, my friend, an everyday—
A livable death at last.

II

*Under Buzzards*

[for Robert Penn Warren]

Heavy summer. Heavy. Companion, if we climb our mortal bodies
High with great effort, we shall find ourselves
Flying with the life
Of the birds of death. We have come up
Under buzzards    they face us

Slowly    slowly circling    and as we watch them they turn us
Around, and you and I spin
Slowly, slowly rounding
Out the hill. We are level
Exactly on this moment: exactly on the same bird-

plane with those deaths. They are the salvation of our sense
Of glorious movement. Brother, it is right for us to face
Them every which way, and come to ourselves and come
From every direction
There is. Whirl and stand fast!
Whence cometh death, O Lord?
On the downwind, riding fire,

Of Hogback Ridge.
But listen: what is dead here?
They are not falling but waiting    but waiting
Riding, and they may know
The rotten, nervous sweetness of my blood.
Somewhere riding the updraft
Of a far forest fire, they sensed the city sugar
The doctors found in time.
My eyes are green as lettuce with my diet,
My weight is down,
One pocket nailed with needles and injections, the other dragging
With sugar cubes to balance me in life
And hold my blood
Level, level. Tell me, black riders, does this do any good?
Tell me what I need to know about my time
In the world. O out of the fiery

Furnace of pine-woods, in the sap-smoke and crownfire of needles,
Say when I'll die. When will the sugar rise boiling
Against me, and my brain be sweetened
to death?
*In heavy summer, like this day.*
All right! Physicians, witness! I will shoot my veins
Full of insulin. Let the needle burn
In. From your terrible heads
The flight-blood drains    and you are falling back
Back to the body-raising

Fire.
Heavy summer. Heavy. My blood is clear
For a time. Is it too clear? Heat waves are rising
Without birds. But something is gone from me,
Friend. This is too sensible. Really it is better
To know when to die    better for my blood
To stream with the death-wish of birds.
You know, I had just as soon crush
This doomed syringe
Between two mountain rocks, and bury this needle in needles

Of trees. Companion, open that beer.
How the body works    how hard it works
For its medical books is not
Everything: everything is how
Much glory is in it: heavy summer is right

For a long drink of beer. Red sugar of my eyeballs
Feels them turn blindly
In the fire    rising    turning    turning
Back to Hogback Ridge, and it is all
Delicious, brother: my body is turning    is flashing unbalanced
Sweetness everywhere, and I am calling my birds.

## The Cost of Appearances
Arthur Frank

Society praises ill persons with words such as "courageous," "optimistic," and "cheerful." Family and friends speak approvingly of the patient who jokes or just smiles, making them, the visitors, feel good. Everyone around the ill person becomes committed to the idea that recovery is the only outcome worth thinking about. No matter what the actual odds, an attitude of "You're going to be fine" dominates the sickroom. Everyone works to sustain it. But how much work does the ill person have to do to make others feel good?

Two kinds of emotional work are involved in being ill. One kind I have written about takes place when the ill person, alone or with true caregivers, works with the emotions of fear, frustration, and loss and tries to find some coherence about what it means to be ill. The other kind is the work the ill person does to keep up an appearance. This appearance is the expectation that a society of healthy friends, coworkers, medical staff, and others places on an ill person.

The appearance most praised is "I'd hardly have known she was sick." At home the ill person must appear to be engaged in normal family routines; in the hospital she should appear to be just resting. When the ill person can no longer conceal the effects of illness, she is expected to convince others that being ill isn't that bad. The minimal acceptable behavior is praised, faintly, as "stoical." But the ill person may not feel like acting good-humored and positive; much of the time it takes hard work to hold this appearance in place.

I have never heard an ill person praised for how well she expressed fear or grief or was openly sad. On the contrary, ill persons feel a need to apologize if they show any emotions other than laughter. Occasional tears may be passed off as the ill person's need to "let go"; the tears are categorized as temporary outbursts instead of understood as part of an ongoing emotion. Sustained "negative" emotions are out of place. If a patient shows too much sadness, he must be depressed, and "depression" is a treatable medical disease.

Too few people, whether medical staff, family, or friends, seem willing to accept the possibility that depression may be the ill person's most appropriate response to the situation. I am not recommending depression, but I do want to suggest that at some moments even fairly deep depression must be accepted as part of the experience of illness.

A couple of days before my mother-in-law died, she shared a room with a woman who was also being treated for cancer. My mother-in-law was this woman's second dying roommate, and the woman was seriously ill herself. I have no doubt that her diagnosis of clinical depression was accurate. The issue is how the medical staff responded to her depression. Instead of trying to understand it as a reasonable response to her situation, her doctors treated her with antidepressant drugs. When a hospital psychologist came to visit her, his questions were designed only to evaluate her "mental status." What day is it? Where are you and what floor are you on? Who is prime minister? and so forth. His sole interest was whether the dosage of antidepressant drug was too high, upsetting her "cognitive orientation." The hospital needed her to be mentally competent so she would remain a "good patient" requiring little extra care; it did not need her emotions. No one attempted to explore her fears with her. No one asked what it was like to have two roommates die within a couple of days of each other, and how this affected her own fear of death. No one was willing to witness her experience.

What makes me saddest is seeing the work ill persons do to sustain this "cheerful patient" image. A close friend of ours, dying of cancer, seriously wondered how her condition could be getting worse, since she had brought homemade cookies to the treatment center whenever she had chemotherapy. She believed there had to be a causal connection between attitude and physical improvement. From early childhood on we are taught that attitude and effort count. "Good citizenship" is supposed to bring us extra points. The nurses all said what a wonderful woman our friend was. She was the perfectly brave, positive, cheerful cancer patient. To me she was most wonderful at the end, when she grieved her illness openly, dropped her act, and clearly demonstrated her anger. She lived her illness as she chose, and by the time she was acting on her anger and sadness, she was too sick for me to ask her if she wished she had expressed more of those emotions earlier. I can only wonder what it had cost her to sustain her happy image for so long.

When I tried to sustain a cheerful and tidy image, it cost me energy, which was scarce. It also cost me opportunities to express what *was* happening in my life with cancer and to understand that life. Finally, my attempts at a positive image diminished my relationships with others by preventing them from sharing my experience. But this image is all that many of those around an ill person are willing to see.

The other side of sustaining a "positive" image is denying that illness can end in death. Medical staff argue that patients who need to deny dying should be allowed to do so. The sad end of this process comes when the person is dying but has become too sick to express what he might now want to say to his loved ones, about his life and theirs. Then that person and his family are denied a final experience together; not all will choose this moment, but all have a right to it.

The medical staff do not have to be part of the tragedy of living with what was left unsaid. For them a patient who denies is one who is cheerful, makes few demands, and asks fewer questions. Some ill persons may need to deny, for reasons we cannot know. But it is too convenient for treatment providers to assume that the denial comes entirely from the patient, because this allows them not to recognize that they are cueing the patient. Labeling the ill person's behavior as denial describes it as a need of the patient, instead of understanding it as the patient's *response* to his situation. That situation, made up of the cues given by treatment providers and caregivers, is what shapes the ill person's behavior.

To be ill is to be dependent on medical staff, family, and friends. Since all these people value cheerfulness, the ill must summon up their energies to be cheerful. Denial may not be what they want or need, but it is what they perceive those around them wanting and needing. This is not the ill person's own denial, but rather his accommodation to the denial of others. When others around you are denying what is happening to you, denying it yourself can seem like your best deal.

To live among others is to make deals. We have to decide what support we need and what we must give others to get that support. Then we make our "best deal" of behavior to get what we need. This process is rarely a conscious one. It develops over a long time in so many experiences that it becomes the way we are, or what we call our personality. But behind much of what we call personality, deals are being made. In a crisis such as illness the terms of the deal rise to the surface and can be seen more clearly.

One incident can stand for all the deals I made during treatment. During my chemotherapy I had to spend three-day periods as an inpatient, receiving continuous drugs. In the three weeks or so between treatments I was examined weekly in the day-care part of the cancer center. Day care is a large room filled with easy chairs where patients sit while they are given briefer intravenous chemotherapy than mine. There are also beds, closely spaced with curtains between. Everyone can see everyone else and hear most of what is being said. Hospitals, however, depend on a myth of privacy. As soon as a curtain is pulled, that space is defined as private, and the patient is expected to answer all questions, no matter how intimate. The first time we went to day care, a young nurse interviewed Cathie and me to assess our "psychosocial" needs. In the middle of this medical bus station she began asking some reasonable questions. Were we experiencing difficulties at work because of my illness? Were we having any problems with our families? Were we getting support from them? These questions were precisely what a caregiver should ask. The problem was where they were being asked.

Our response to most of these questions was to lie. Without even looking at each other, we both understood that whatever problems we were having, we were not going to talk about them there. Why? To figure out our best deal, we had to assess the kind of support we thought we could get in that setting from that nurse. Nothing she did convinced us that what she could offer was equal to what we would risk by telling her the truth.

Admitting that you have problems makes you vulnerable, but it is also the only way to get help. Throughout my illness Cathie and I constantly weighed our need for help against the risk involved in making ourselves vulnerable. If we did not feel that support was forthcoming, we suppressed our need for expression. If we had expressed our problems and emotions in that very public setting, we would have been extremely vulnerable. If we had then received anything less than total support, it would have been devastating. The nurse showed no awareness or appreciation of how much her questions required us to risk, so we gave only a cheerful "no problems" response. That was all the setting seemed able to support.

Maybe we were wrong. Maybe the staff would have supported us if we had opened up our problems with others' responses to my illness, our stress trying to keep our jobs going, and our fears and doubts about treatment. We certainly were aware that our responses cut off that support. It was double or nothing; we chose safety. Ill persons face such choices constantly. We still believe we were right to keep quiet. If the staff had had real support to offer, they would have offered it in a setting that encouraged our response. When we were alone with nurses in an inpatient room, the questions they asked were those on medical history forms. In the privacy of that room the nurses were vulnerable to the emotions we might have expressed, so they asked no "psychosocial" questions.

It was a lot of work for us to answer the day-care nurse's questions with a smile. Giving her the impression that we felt all right was draining, and illness and its care had drained us both already. But expending our energies this way seemed our best deal.

Anybody who wants to be a caregiver, particularly a professional, must not only have real support to offer but must also learn to convince the ill person that this support is there. My defenses have never been stronger than they were when I was ill. I have never watched others more closely or been more guarded around them. I needed others more than I ever have, and I was also most vulnerable to them. The behavior I worked to let others see was my most conservative estimate of what I thought they would support.

Again I can give no formula, only questions. To the ill person: How much is this best deal costing you in terms of emotional work? What are you compromising of your own expression of illness in order to present those around you with the cheerful appearance they want? What do you fear will happen if you act otherwise? And to those around the ill person: What cues are you giving the ill person that tell her how you want her to act? In what way is her behavior a response to your own? Whose denial, whose needs?

Fear and depression are a part of life. In illness there are no "negative emotions," only experiences that have to be lived through. What is needed in these moments is not denial but recognition. The ill person's suffering should be affirmed, whether or not it can be treated. What I wanted when I was most ill was the response, "Yes, we see your pain; we accept your fear." I needed others to recognize not only that I was suffering, but also that we had this suffering in common. I can accept that doctors and nurses sometimes fail to provide the correct treatment. But I cannot accept it when medical staff, family, and friends fail to recognize that they are equal participants in the process of illness. Their actions shape the behavior of the ill person, and their bodies share the potential of illness.

Those who make cheerfulness and bravery the price they require for support deny their own humanity. They deny that to be human is to be mortal, to become ill and die. Ill persons need others to share in recognizing with them the frailty of the human body. When others join the ill person in this recognition, courage and cheer may be the result, not as an appearance to be worked at, but as a spontaneous expression of a common emotion.

**Betting Your Life**
Alice Stewart Trillin

Jerome Groopman has written about the dilemma a doctor faces when giving medical advice that strongly contradicts the diagnosis of another doctor, and about the difficulty of waiting rather than taking swift action in the face of a dire medical situation. He recalled an admonition he heard as a medical student: "Don't just do something—stand there." But what about a patient who has to bet his life on one doctor's best guess against another's, and stands there, waiting to see which way the possibly loaded dice will roll?

In September of 1990, my husband and I took a trip to Istanbul. A few days before we left, I came down with a case of what my internist took to be flu, but not a serious enough case to make me cancel the trip. Yet, after the long plane flight and a few days breathing Istanbul's polluted air, I couldn't stop coughing. Fourteen years earlier, I'd been diagnosed with lung cancer—I was thirty-eight and had never smoked—and had a lobe of my left lung removed, followed by radiation and some chemotherapy. I'd been well since then, and had finally come to believe that this particular cancer probably wouldn't kill me; it certainly didn't occur to me that my cough was anything more than an annoying symptom of the flu. But when, back in New York, I went to see an oncologist at Memorial Sloan-Kettering Cancer Center for a checkup, a chest X-ray showed fluid inside the lower lining of each of my lungs—bilateral pleural effusions. The oncologist was worried enough about what this might mean to schedule a needle aspiration of the fluid for the next day.

Bending over a table as a doctor inserted a needle into my back to extract some fluid, I started to think about what I would do if a presumably innocent cough turned out to be the sound of the other shoe dropping. I had once had good reason to listen for that other shoe; I'd had malignant lymph nodes in my mediastinum—the middle of my chest—as well as a tumor in my lung. I had always been amazed at how little time I'd spent listening for it, and what I most disliked about having the needle stuck into my back was that it began to awaken what I'd come to think of as the dragon that sleeps inside anyone who has had cancer. I'd written once that we can never kill this dragon, but we go about the business of our daily lives—giving our children breakfast, putting more mulch on our gardens—in the hope that it will stay asleep for a while longer. What I hadn't said was what I'd do if the dragon woke up. But, even as I braced myself for the insertion of the needle, it seemed unlikely that lung cancer, a notoriously aggressive disease, would hang around for so long only to reassert itself in the guise of a cough that interfered with my dreams of seeing the Bosporus.

A biopsy of the fluid showed no suspicious cells. The doctors called it inconclusive, because it could have been a false negative. My two daughters were coming home for the Christmas holidays, so I tried not to think about why I still couldn't stop coughing. Then, early in January, I suddenly felt a sharp pain in my back, which I assumed was a result of irritation caused by the pleural effusions. When it didn't go away, I had another chest X-ray, and that was when the dragon started breathing smoke. The X-ray, I was told, showed what appeared to be a fracture in one of the vertebrae in my thoracic spine—the part of the spine that lies over the lungs—and soon afterward I got a call from Kathleen Foley, a neurologist at Memorial who had become a friend over the years. My regular oncologist was away, and I had asked Kathy to look at the X-ray. She was concerned about the fracture, and ordered an MRI for the next day. I have come to hate MRIs, and as I lay inside the tomblike steel tube I started, finally, to get really scared.

The MRI looked "funny" to the doctors who read it, and when Kathy called with the results I knew that I was in trouble. When I asked her what the MRI might mean, she was, as always, both gentle and completely honest.

"It might be a tumor. That's what we're most worried about. That's what it looks like to the radiologist."

I asked her if it could be anything else.

"Well, yes, it might be a relatively rare infection of the bone, but it's unlikely you'd have that."

"O.K.," I said. "What do we do now?"

She told me, unequivocally, what we were going to do. It was a Friday—does all bad medical news come on a Friday?—and she'd already begun to schedule a series of tests, beginning at eight Monday morning. First, I would have a needle biopsy of the suspicious vertebra. Then I'd have a bone scan. By the end of the day, we should know something definitive. We agreed that the best course was to act quickly, because for me not knowing what is going on in my body is far worse than any awful certainty that might be discovered. My imagination can always conjure up images that are scarier than any produced by an X-ray machine. At least, that's what I'd thought until Monday afternoon, when Kathy slapped my bone scan onto the panel above her desk and flipped on the light behind it.

Kathleen Foley is a handsome woman, then in her late forties, slim and graceful, with stylishly cut gray-blond hair. She usually wears the standard female-doctor outfit—white coat over neat blouse, straight skirt, sensible pumps—but she carries it in a way that suggests a closetful of really good clothes at home. Her manner is straightforward and professional, but she laughs easily and lets you know right away that she will listen carefully to everything you say. I had met Kathy following a medical scare not long after my surgery. Looking down to sign a hotel register, I had felt a spasm like an electric current move along my back from the base of my skull to my toes. Every time I repeated the movement, the spasm recurred. That was the other shoe, for sure. (Likely metastatic sites for lung cancer are the brain and the spine.) I spent the week trying not to tell my husband what I thought was happening. When I got home, I was referred to Kathy, as much because my oncologist knew that we would like each other as because she had a reputation as an outstanding young neurologist. I met her on a Monday morning, and by that afternoon she was able to tell me that I had something called Lhermitte's Sign, a not unusual side effect of radiation to the chest.

When I saw her a year later, my best friend was dying of kidney cancer and I, who had never had a headache in my life, suddenly found myself with a pounding pain at the top of my skull. After a "just to rule out the worst" X-ray, Kathy diagnosed tooth grinding as the cause, and told me how tense she had been recently when she was away for too long from her two young boys, who were about the same age as my girls. Years later, one of my daughters and one of her sons found themselves living down the hall from each other at college, and Kathy and I had become good friends.

Kathy said later that she wished she had looked at the bone scan before showing it to me and my husband, and that she would have if she hadn't known me as well as she did. She understood that I wanted to know the truth, but neither she nor I anticipated what it would be like when we all looked at five "lights" that showed up on the bone scan—two in my ribs, two in my hips, and one in my spine. Each light indicated a possible tumor.

"What do you think it is?" I asked.

She told me that, if she had to guess, she'd say it was a late metastasis to the bone, from my lung cancer. Unlikely, but not impossible. Of course, there might be other explanations, though she couldn't think of any at the time. The important thing, as always, was to move fast and try not to think too much about what to do if none of the aggressive tactics worked. That's what I'd done fourteen years before—I'd coughed up a tiny blood clot, seen my doctor immediately, and had a lobe of my lung removed ten days later. I didn't have second opinions, I didn't agonize over the decision. That's what I always told the people who called me for advice when they found out they had cancer. Serious medical decisions are not philosophical decisions; X-rays and scans and biopsies are the key; science will tell you what to do.

At eight the next morning, I checked into Memorial's day hospital, a surprisingly pleasant place on the seventeenth floor of an imposing building on Manhattan's Upper East Side. Memorial had terrified me when I first walked in the door, years earlier, but I had somehow come to feel comfortable and safe there. (I began to like the place on that first day, when a young man with no hair—a leukemia patient—asked what was wrong with me. When I mumbled "lung cancer," he smiled and said, "They treat that like the common cold around here.") Kathy came to see me early, and told me that she'd been thinking about my scan and thought there might be some other explanation for what was going on, possibly something having to do with my radiation. I wrote that off as an attempt to cheer me up. The biopsy of the vertebra that I'd had the day before was also inconclusive, so the radiologist spent the morning trying to get a better specimen—one that would show just what kind of tumor might be eating up my spine. I lay on my stomach for most of the morning, moving in and out of a CAT scanner, trying to use techniques I vaguely remembered from natural-childbirth classes to doze through the numerous probes. At the end of the day, we still had no conclusive results, and Kathy scheduled a consultation for me with a neurosurgeon at Memorial. We had to consider the possibility that the only way we would find out what the shadow on my spine meant was to take it out.

I am known among my friends and family as an incorrigible, even ridiculous optimist. I think all optimists fear that one day they will wake up and won't be able to put a hopeful spin on anything ever again. This is what happened to my father, who was known for an optimism that got him through years of bankruptcies and disappointments, and which vanished like dust when my mother had Alzheimer's.

In the days after that bone scan, I couldn't find a hopeful way out of what those lights seemed to tell me. I did manage to imagine uplifting conversations I might have with my daughters about how it was OK for me to die this time, as it absolutely had not been when they were four and seven, and I had foreseen their adoring but occasionally absent-minded father getting them the wrong kind of sneakers or losing track of their dental appointments after I was gone. Now one of them was in college, and the other was teaching in California, and I was sure that I had told them everything of importance I knew; they had understood it all and figured out a lot on their own, and were as close to perfect as they could possibly be. Then it occurred to me that neither of them was married yet, and I would hate to miss the weddings and the grandchildren. I speculated about which of my friends I would assign to help them pick out their wedding dresses. Then I cried and decided that I really wanted to stay around, particularly when I started to think about the women who might come after my husband when I was gone. (The best description of this feeling came from my friend Josie Mankewitz Davis, who died young in a traffic accident, and who had said to her husband, years earlier, that if anything happened to her she'd certainly expect him to marry again, particularly because he would need help raising their children. Then she paused for a beat, and added, "Just don't sleep with her!")

I continued to move fast. I saw the neurosurgeon Kathy had recommended, who looked at the MRI and urged me to have surgery immediately, so that he could remove the suspicious vertebra and replace it with a steel rod. He couldn't be sure that what he saw was cancer, but clearly he suspected that it was. In a year or so, if the tumor hadn't turned out to be malignant, he would operate again and replace the rod with a piece of bone from my leg. Each of these surgeries would involve a thoracotomy—my spine would be reached through a large incision in my chest—because my back was too scarred by radiation to allow a successful incision. In other words, I would be taken apart twice in one year if I was lucky enough not to have cancer, with about a 30% chance of infection (because of the extensive radiation scarring) and a chance of permanent damage to my back each time. On the other hand, this course offered certainty; at least, we'd know what was in there. For the first time in my life, the idea of medical certainty had lost its appeal.

Then, three days after the bone scan, I was offered a fragile rope with which I could begin to pull myself out of the tunnel I felt I'd been living in. I was getting an X-ray of a rib where one of the suspicious lights had appeared, in preparation for yet another bone biopsy, when the radiologist hurried into the room and said to me, "Have you fallen lately?" I hadn't, and I asked him why this was relevant; he said that, much to his surprise, the lesion in my rib looked more like a fracture than like a tumor. At that moment, I felt a physical rush—perhaps my recently vanished optimism was flowing back into my body. If this lesion in my rib might not be a tumor, what about the other suspicious bone sites?

Kathy was ecstatic, and together we started planning the next step. I thought of us as a tiny Amazon army, with Kathy as the general, and me following her directions as we looked for reinforcements. First, she sent me to see another neurosurgeon, a famous technician at another hospital. He didn't think it was necessary to examine me, but he told me that even though he couldn't be sure that my MRI revealed cancer, he was sure that my spine would soon collapse if I didn't have surgery. He also said that I should begin wearing a back brace immediately, and take taxis everywhere if I absolutely had to leave the house, because if I fell I might sever my spine and become a paraplegic. Not having seen the radiation scarring, he suggested that he operate as soon as possible, through my back.

Surgery had saved my life once before, and I liked the idea of getting rid of whatever was in my spine. There was nothing more we could learn from the technology of medicine; we had done all the tests that could reasonably be done, and none had given us a definitive answer. Despite the ambiguous X-ray of my rib, the surgeons and the radiologists I'd consulted all agreed that I should act right away. But there had been something unsatisfying about my conversations with them; Kathy and I decided to seek a few more medical opinions before deciding what to do.

Most of the many words that have been written about "doctor-patient communication" have come from doctors; there are textbooks devoted to the subject, and communication "competencies" are now taught in a number of medical schools. It would be difficult for me to come up with a list of competencies I look for in a doctor, but I know when I have met one I will trust. Mark Kris, who heads the thoracic-oncology service at Memorial, was this kind of doctor. Kathy sent me to see him for the same reasons I'd been sent to her years before—because he was brilliant, and because she knew I'd like him. The first thing Mark did, after looking at my medical records and having me carefully retell the story of what had happened to me over the past few months, was to give me a thorough examination. This was the first physical I'd had since this drama began; everyone else had just looked at the X-rays and scans. After he finished, he asked me how I felt. It was the only time in these months that anyone had asked me that question.

"I feel fine, except for a pretty severe pain in my back."

"You look really well, too," Mark said. A woman is always happy to hear this, especially from an attractive man, but I took what he said as another attempt to cheer me up.

"Well, I looked pretty good, and felt fine, too, when I had lung cancer," I said.

He looked at me intently. "Yes, but this is different. If you had widely metastasized cancer, as the MRI and scans seem to suggest, you shouldn't feel this well, or look this well, either." This was not a compliment; it was a diagnosis.

"Do you mean you think this might not be cancer?" I asked skeptically.

"I honestly don't know, but I'm not sure that it is, and my advice is that you give this some time, if you can stand it, and see how this develops."

I couldn't believe what I was hearing, or what I was feeling. A very smart doctor was asking me to live with the possibility that I might have five tumors growing in my bones, and to do nothing but wait and watch. The advice went against everything I'd come to believe about acting aggressively to fight cancer. But it made sense to me. I had one more question for Mark.

"What if it is cancer?"

He paused, thinking hard about what to say. "If it is, you will come back to me and I will tell you what we can do. I will also tell you what I think you should do, and then you can make up your mind."

That did it. That was when I knew I would trust this man. He had understood exactly what my question meant. I had been thinking about whether, if I did have metastatic lung cancer, I would do anything at all. Sometimes doctor-patient communication doesn't have to rely on words.

I had one more doctor to see before we made our decision: Joseph Lane, an orthopedist and bone specialist, who practiced at Memorial and at the Hospital for Special Surgery, across the street. He was known both for his brusqueness and for his diagnostic skill, and he saw so many patients that I was prepared for a long wait and a short audience. After spending about five hours in the Memorial waiting room, my husband and I were taken to a small examining room, where I changed into the ubiquitous hospital gown, and we waited some more. Finally, a parade of white coats rushed into the room, led by a short, energetic man whom my husband later described as having the manner of "a salesman for Nobody Beats the Wiz," followed by Kathy Foley, who was carrying my medical records. Dr. Lane reviewed them quickly, and then checked my back and chest for radiation damage, noting a tiny tattoo that marked the focal point of my radiation, just above the fractured vertebra. His words came in bursts: "Nope, this doesn't look like tumor to me. Radiation necrosis—a lot of that now in women radiated for breast cancer. Not so much in lung cancer, not that many live long enough." The white coats dutifully took notes. I had almost lost the ability to speak, but I managed to ask him what he thought I should do. "We'll put you on calcitonin—it works for about eighteen months. You inject yourself three times a week—strengthens the bones. Have an MRI every month or so for a year to see if anything else shows up. Take calcium, and a multivitamin to support the calcium. Nope, definitely not tumor."

My husband spoke for the first time: "You're our favorite doctor so far." All I could think to ask was what kind of vitamin I should take.

Dr. Lane seemed to consider this seriously. "El cheapo is el besto," he answered with a grin, as if he had just closed the deal on a color television.

"OK," I said, feeling as if he'd just prescribed a newly discovered monoclonal antibody or breakthrough gene therapy. He wished me good luck and breezed out of the room, followed closely by his disciples. Not exactly a conventional model for the doctor-patient communication textbooks, but effective all the same.

After I got a shot of calcitonin from Dr. Lane's nurse—the first therapeutic action I'd taken since all this began—my husband and I drove home to Greenwich Village, unable to say anything for a while. Then we heard on the radio that the Gulf War seemed to be ending, and we remembered that the lights in my bone scan had shown up on the very day that the fighting in Iraq had begun. Could this be it? Could our own Gulf War end up being, like my Lhermitte's scare of years ago, just part of the price I paid for the five thousand rads of cobalt that may have saved my life? Was this turning out to be not tragedy but farce, with a Nobody Beats the Wiz salesman as the comic deus ex machina?

Jerome Groopman writes that "human biology is too variable to be reduced to mathematical calculation. Intuition would still count, and so would luck." As we drove down the East Side Drive, my husband pointed out that none of the facts—the "mathematical calculations"—had changed since that first terrifying set of test results. All the contradictory advice we'd got had been based on the same information. Why were we now willing to place our bets on Mark Kris and Joseph Lane, and not on the surgeons and the radiologists we had talked to? Naturally, I wanted to believe what Mark Kris and Joseph Lane told me, but it was more than that. I also believed them because I trusted them, and because my own intuitions about what was going on in my body told me they might be right. Although I'm not sure I understood this at the time, I now think I trusted them because they were able to see the mathematical calculations of my case in a wider context than the surgeons and the radiologists had. Mark Kris had seen thousands of patients with lung cancer, and there was something about my symptoms and appearance that made him question the diagnosis of metastatic disease. Similarly, Joseph Lane routinely saw cases of radiation necrosis, and the shadows in my bones were less ominous to him than they had been to others. Even though, like all the other doctors at Memorial, they both saw me as someone who had once had a cancer with a very grim prognosis, they were able to look beyond this prognosis for another cause of my symptoms. And, by providing context, they helped me widen the lens through which I viewed what was happening to me. They gave me the courage to wait. Of course, they might have been wrong.

A year later, it appeared that they hadn't been. It was generally agreed that my vertebra had collapsed as the result of radiation necrosis and probably wouldn't move far enough to sever my spine; my ribs had broken mysteriously, possibly because of violent coughing, but were healing nicely; the lights in my hips probably showed age-related arthritis; and the pleural effusions had been a result of the flu. The dragon had gone back to sleep for a while longer. Almost ten years have passed. One of my daughters got married last summer, and the other will be married in May. I helped them pick out their dresses.

# The Want of Control: Ideas and Ideals in the Management of Diabetes

Chris Feudtner

Better treatment of diabetes should be universal. Diabetes should be controlled. The means are at our door.—Elliott P. Joslin, "A Renaissance of the Control of Diabetes," 1954

In the early spring of 1927, four-year-old Arnold Burns arrived in Boston. A month previous, consumed by an unslakable thirst and a boundless appetite, he had begun to urinate frequently. His local doctor, upon finding sugar in Arnold's urine, immediately referred the boy and his mother, Ethel Burns, to the Joslin Clinic. After traveling the 50 miles from their Massachusetts home to Boston, Arnold was seen by Dr. Priscilla White, a 27-year-old member of the clinic staff who was in charge of juvenile cases. She noted that the child was frail and "drowsy," breathing deeply but otherwise "normal."[1] Once Arnold was admitted to the hospital, he and his mother spent a week learning about diabetes and how to control it through assiduous home management. Upon his departure from Boston, no longer healthy or carefree, he was required (with his mother's help) to inject three doses of insulin each day and follow a diet of precisely 960 calories.[2]

This rigorous style of managing diabetic life was exactly what Elliott Joslin envisioned as ideal care. Joslin believed in patient education and self-control even before he first administered insulin in 1922. Now, with the aid of the wondrous drug, he felt that disciplined diabetics could attain mastery over their disease. In this unabashedly assured spirit, Joslin wrote to the boy's local doctor a fortnight after Arnold was discharged. "Anything I can do to help you with that Burns case," he declared, "would be

Chris Feudtner, "The Want of Control: Ideas and Ideals in the Management of Diabetes," from *Bittersweet: Diabetes, Insulin, and the Transformation of Illness*, 121–145. © 2003 by the University of North Carolina Press. Reprinted by permission of the publisher.

a pleasure. Of course you know that these diabetic children under ten years of age formerly died at an average duration of less than 1 [year] and 2 tenths, but now they appear to live indefinitely."[3] Like the majority of his medical colleagues, Joslin was confident that insulin had rewritten the future of the once swiftly fatal juvenile diabetes.

And so it had. Patients like Arnold survived well beyond childhood—but they certainly did not survive indefinitely. As insulin entered the clinical scene, no one suspected that the history of diabetes would become a story juxtaposing "success" and "failure" as a perceived medical victory evolved into an ambiguous and frustrating clinical reality. No one foresaw that many diabetic patients, while surviving longer, would be beset by painful or debilitating complications before succumbing to an unpleasant death. No one predicted the problems that transmuted diabetes would bring to the lives of patients.

The resulting intellectual and emotional dialectic—between triumphal and tragic outlooks—has long animated diabetic therapeutics, driving it almost obsessively toward the alluring yet elusive goal of controlling the course of disease.[4] Simply put, the modern medical management of diabetes mellitus has been shaped by four often contradictory ideals: complete cure, constant regulation, physician control, and patient control. These ideals, when put into practice, have generated tensions that have shaped the lives of diabetics, their families, and their doctors—who, importantly, have disagreed among themselves as to the health consequences of "tight" or "poor" diabetic control. Therefore the human dimensions of the transformation of diabetes, spurred by a series of remarkable technical innovations, can best be understood by exploring how these ideals have been made manifest in thought and action.[5]

These shifts of biological process and therapeutic style have embedded the specific care of any given diabetic patient within a broader historical process, as prevailing ideas, innovations, and ideals have combined around the circumstances of a personal history, medical and otherwise. These components—specific individual experiences and general historical patterns—are inextricably connected and are best viewed as essentially complementary silhouettes of each other: the individual experiences compose the broader patterns, which in turn shape the individual experiences. Consequently, a historical overview of diabetic management must strive for a balance in its narrative account between this yin and yang, situating seemingly idiosyncratic occurrences and choices into the wider context of historical trends within a society and its cultural and social arrangements, using each aspect to explain the other.

### Insulin and Control "among the Erstwhile Dead"

The introduction of insulin in 1922 seemed to mark a sharp break with past therapeutic practices, providing physicians with a drug of unprecedented power and efficacy. Insulin also appeared to validate the "pancreatic theory" of diabetes. Based largely upon Minkowski and von Mering's creation of diabetes in dogs by resection of their pancreases and Opie's pathological studies of diabetic pancreases devoid of islets of Langerhans, the pancreatic theory located the cause of diabetes in this organ, spurring investigators to quest for the elusive internal pancreatic secretion.[6] Insulin's dramatic effects seemed unassailable proof that these ideas were essentially correct; the fundamental problem was too little insulin from the pancreas. Reasoning by analogy to the treatment of hypothyroidism (myxedema) with thyroid gland extract, many enthusiasts thought that insulin was about to convert treated diabetes into a benign entity. Even if insulin would not produce a radical cure, this form of organotherapy would prove nevertheless to be an extraordinarily effective specific treatment.

But insulin did more than support medical theories and enable patients to metabolize food. This potent medical innovation and the surrounding network of ideas, in the mind of Joslin and many other physicians, subtly reconfigured therapeutic ideals. The conquest of all diabetic complications—a medical campaign that Joslin had mapped out in his Shattuck Lecture, delivered before the Massachusetts Medical Society in the spring of 1922—became a new composite ideal. The aims of treatment began to move through the framework of constant and meticulous regulation (now aided by insulin) toward the complete cure of all untoward consequences of being diabetic. Two years after insulin was first put into use, Joslin enthused that "a new race of diabetics has come upon the scene." The Nobel Prize–winning discovery by Banting, Best, Collip, and Macleod had already extended the lives of diabetics by two years; "hospital practice, therefore," Joslin continued, "this past year has been among the erstwhile dead."[7] Not that Joslin viewed the extract as a panacea: "insulin does not cure diabetes," he stated repeatedly.[8] But, with insulin in hand to complement diet and exercise, he and his collaborators seemed to think that all manifestations of the disease (except the need to care constantly for oneself) could and should be eliminated.[9]

Patients such as Arnold Burns were the first generation after insulin to be indoctrinated in these values of intensive regulatory control. When Arnold was admitted to the Joslin Clinic and spent a week in the hospital, he and his mother, Ethel, learned about his disease and the proper use of diet and insulin. Such an experience was exactly what Joslin, from the pulpit of his self-styled diabetic care movement, had spelled out as ideal care, a high road to total mastery of the disease.

In Arnold's case, the early lessons of care and control were overseen at the Joslin Clinic by Dr. Priscilla White, who had joined Joslin's staff in 1924. White attended to juvenile patients and their parents throughout her distinguished career. She wrote a groundbreaking monograph, *Diabetes in Childhood and Adolescence* (1932), and was a pioneer in the field of prenatal care for pregnant diabetic women and their babies. Although herself a proselytizer of Joslin's doctrine of control, numerous sources (from journal articles and correspondence to anecdotes and testimonials) indicate that she delivered the message to patients in a distinct style, tempered with personal warmth, imbued with almost "charismatic attention" and concern. "No child," she believed, "can grow up without a scoop of ice cream once a week."[10]

Even Joslin—whose professional enthusiasm for diabetic control led some of his contemporaries to view him as an overly demanding zealot— also spoke to patients in more flexible and understanding registers, enunciating facts of diabetic life in soothing tones. In published works and private letters, Joslin often dwelled upon the mundane realities of living with diabetes. His therapeutics often consisted of simple advice, comprehensive in scope, delivered with the assured certainty of an experienced general practitioner who was comfortable managing many areas of patients' lives.

For example, after one of Arnold's visits to the clinic, Joslin conveyed to Mrs. Burns that young Arnold was developing normally both physically and mentally. He then went on to suggest that the boy's mildly protuberant abdomen might be helped by gentle exercises and that he should be "out in the sun as much as possible, should take cod liver oil, a teaspoonful daily, and eat liver twice a week in place of his usual meat."[11]

On another occasion, Ethel wrote Joslin that she was "taking advantage of the fact that you said I might write and ask you any question. I would like to know how to treat a cough? Arnold developed a cold and cough. . . .

He has several coughs like this every winter and Arnold's father feels I have failed in my duty not to have asked you before now what to do." She had heard Joslin say that "codeine was the medicine a mother would give when you spoke over Radio about 2 yrs ago so I bought some Codeine . . . and it worked very well[;] now I would like to know if that was right? Arnold [is] fine now."[12] Joslin quickly replied that he thought the codeine unnecessary. "Upon just placing a child in bed," he advised, "with the quiet which that implies or either some tablet or even chewing gum, the cough should subside." Closing his note, he added: "We are always glad to answer questions."[13]

From bulging bellies to troublesome coughs to constipated bowels, Joslin had advice to dispense. Frequently, though, his patients presented more complex and often competing needs, many of which revolved around financial constraints that eroded patients' ability to control their disease. The medical records of his clinic are filled with references to money problems exacerbated by the burdens of buying insulin and other diabetic medical care.[14]

Arnold's mother referred frequently to money and costs. Once, she inquired about a bill that the clinic had sent for a pediatrician's examination that had taken place when she had last brought Arnold to the clinic. She explained, "It has puzzled me as to why [the pediatrician] was called in and nothing said until afterward. We are perfectly willing to do all that is necessary to help Arnold but we are not financially able to do anything that is not necessary and I am writing this so we'll understand each others['] ways." Having reasserted her prerogative to control how her family would spend money on Arnold's medical care, she closed by adding, "I hope you will understand the principle of this letter."[15] Three years later, she told Joslin that a year and a half had passed since she "last had Arnold to see you[;] since that time, owing to financial reasons, I have had to take 'a chance' with him that everything was alright."[16]

Things went from bad to worse for the Burns family when Arnold's father died suddenly from a stroke.[17] A month later, Ethel turned to Joslin for help. "Do you happen to have a woman patient," she wrote, "who would like to live in the country by any chance? I am desperate and must find a way to make a little money to help keep Arnold going as he should. . . . I would not bother to ask you if it were not that I must do something and am trying every way I can think of."[18] Although Arnold's medical file does not record what solution Ethel eventually found, clearly this case and similar ones impressed Joslin. Throughout his career, he

solicited money to establish hospital charity funds and advocated medical care cost reform, and when confronted with a patient who could not
pay, he frequently waived his fees and pressured his colleagues to do
likewise.[19]

Money, however, was not the only factor shaping Arnold's health care.
His insulin-transformed disease was still a lurking nemesis that physicians, now with emboldened expectations, sought to subdue through better control. Arnold lived as one of the "erstwhile dead," a young diabetic
always threatened by lethal complications, particularly coma. In the late
1920s, Joslin had spearheaded a campaign to abolish diabetic coma. As he
viewed it, "Diabetes is a chronic disease, but diabetic coma is an acute
disease. If this fact was recognized, deaths from diabetic coma should
cease." The physician had to spot impending coma and treat it vigorously,
while "the patient should be trained to avoid coma." A 1929 editorial in
the *Journal of the American Medical Association* concurred, defining
diabetic coma as "a medical state, possible to prevent, expensive, time
consuming, and difficult to treat, recovery a miracle to all beholders, but
death a lasting blot upon the reputation of the patient or his physician."[20]

Certainly, Joslin knew through his extensive network of correspon-
dents how diabetics had languished or even perished because of poor medical care, such as treating coma with glucose or a host of other needless
mishaps.[21] When Arnold was 11 years old, he nearly suffered a "lasting
blot" upon what would have been his short-lived reputation, but he was
resuscitated at the New England Deaconess Hospital, where his doctors
followed an exacting protocol of treatment with large doses of insulin and
intravenous fluids.[22] After this scare, Priscilla White wrote to Ethel, "Just
why [Arnold] developed diabetic coma I am not certain. Children change
very quickly." White went on,

> A safe program for you to follow on a day of illness would be to test
> the urine every 4 hours, to give 20 units of insulin if the [Benedict's]
> test is red, 15 if the test is orange, 10 units if the test is yellow, 5 units
> if yellow-green. If three consecutive specimens are red give him the
> same amount of insulin only give it every 2 hours instead of every 4
> hours. During the day he could take 1½ quarts of milk, 60 grams of
> bread, 60 grams of potato, 30 grams of oatmeal, 200 grams of orange
> juice or gingerale.[23]

Diabetic coma and its grave consequences warranted this level of precision, since painstaking attention to detail could avert deaths.[24]

Nevertheless, intensive control applied to the daily management of diabetes was the Joslin Clinic's style—not a universal one. For example, the eminent Chicago medical chemist and diabetologist Rollin Turner Woodyatt, MD, who was among the first American physicians to administer insulin, argued for a very different therapeutic strategy to a colleague in 1929. A canny researcher of meticulous habits, drawn more to his laboratory bench than his clinical practice, Woodyatt believed that "the object of treatment is . . . to keep the patient as well and strong as a normal individual with the least effort and with the lowest economic outlay possible, i.e., to make the patient as nearly normal as possible notwithstanding the existence of a nearly total diabetes."[25] Woodyatt, who had developed complex and rather daring dietetic formulas in the pre-insulin era,[26] was willing to concede sugar in diabetic patients' urine in order to avoid insulin reactions. Though Joslin and others were correct in protesting that the urine sugar test then became useless, the point for Woodyatt was moot since he instructed his patients to test their urine for acid and admonished them to stay acid free, not sugar free. In Woodyatt's opinion, the more liberal regimen (he advocated combining regular insulin doses so that there were only two injections a day) allowed a more normal life: "I think it is important with these youngsters in school or college to interfere as little as possible with their free physical, social and psychological development."[27]

But Arnold was a patient under the care of Joslin, not Woodyatt nor any other distinguished physician.[28] For Arnold, debates between experts mattered far less than practical urban-rural differences: living in a small town in rural Massachusetts posed its own problems. Medical knowledge has never been uniformly distributed,[29] and the heterogeneity of clinical experience and practice styles was a prominent aspect of many young diabetics' lives. While elite physicians in Boston felt comfortable dosing insulin and managing diabetic problems, local practitioners were often intimidated by the children's disease.

Ethel related one such incident to White. Shortly after seeing White, who had changed Arnold's diet and insulin, Arnold had broken out in a red rash, with a red throat. Initially, the local doctor had considered scarlet fever to be the cause, but the next day he changed his mind: "He decided it was a re-action to more insulin and different diet. Dr. came again yesterday to just look at throat and wanted me to write to you and tell you all about it and see what you thought, he says he never saw such a violent reaction. He is very interested. . . . Will you please tell me what to do?"[30] Alarmed, White dashed off a note. This might be, she said, a "toxic rash. I am quite worried about [Arnold] and the liberties he has taken with his diet and wish that you could let him come to the hospital for a week. I would be glad to have him come in on one of the funds. There will be no charge for medical care and no charge for the hospital."[31]

Arnold was hurried to the Deaconess Hospital, where the redness of his rash faded and his sore throat improved. White started him on the new, long-acting protamine insulin. Upon returning home, Ethel wrote White that Arnold was "delighted to only have insulin once a day and he is like a different young man he's so interested and bothers so much with his diet and tests. He also shows the good effects by stating he would have liked to have stayed in hospital longer, he was so interested and learning so much." She was pleased, too, that "his diet satisfies so much better and although he gets dizzy and shaky a little mornings he says not as shaky as he was, and straightens with lunch."[32]

### Striving for Control of Life and Death

It was the summer of 1938, and Arnold was 15 years old. Ten years would pass before he contacted Joslin or White again. Like other young diabetics, Arnold was growing up, a member of a cohort of patients new to the world: juvenile-onset diabetics who lived well into adulthood. Many of these patients appeared to be uplifting portraits of therapeutic success; they engaged in competitive athletics, embarked on prestigious careers, bore children, raised families.[33] But for others, this portrait was beginning to be sketched in somber colors. In 1934, the *New England Journal of Medicine* ran an editorial that asked, "Of what shall diabetics die?" While coma and gangrene should no longer be permitted to kill patients, the *Journal* foresaw tuberculosis, pneumonia, stroke, and heart attack as the main causes of death.[34] Two years later, however, Paul Kimmelstiel and Clifford Wilson identified a specific pathologic lesion in the kidneys of diabetics, the first research finding heralding the emergence of renal failure as a major complication for many juvenile-onset diabetics.[35] By the middle of the 1950s, the Joslin Clinic was reporting that 50% of the young patients who died did so in renal failure, many when they were in their thirties.[36] This grim reality unfolded with bitter irony as the transmuted course of diabetes—the product of a singularly efficacious medical innovation—revealed one distressing complication after another.

Arnold reestablished his correspondence with Joslin in the midst of these ominous developments in the early spring of 1948. He was 25 years old and now spoke for himself, having assumed the responsibilities of work with much pride, his sense of self seemingly tied to his mastery of this chronic ailment. "I have been Working for the past six months as an automobile mechanic," he informed Joslin, "and have lost no time due to my diabetes." Then, although it violated one of Joslin's central tenets of ideal routine diabetic care, Arnold declared, "I have been to no doctor in connection to my diabetes since 1939 [nine years ago]."[37] Arnold's mother also recognized her son's pride in his work and his attendance, telling Joslin, "Arnold is getting along very well, . . . and works hard and steady as an auto mechanic, in fact he keeps up with the others not giving in days when I know he'd like to take it easy."[38]

Two years later, Arnold was asked to partake in a clinical study that Howard Root (a senior member of Joslin's staff) and another doctor at the Joslin Clinic were conducting. When Arnold agreed, trouble began to appear, albeit only in abnormal test results. Sugar was spilling into his urine and he had mildly elevated blood pressure, but more ominously, Arnold's eyes showed signs of substantial retinopathy and his kidneys were starting to struggle, with albumin appearing in his urine and an elevated urea level in his blood.[39]

A year and a half passed before these findings manifested themselves clinically. Ethel informed Joslin that she was "writing for Arnold. . . . He is working but acts so very weary, I would like to know what tonic he could take."[40] Several days later, Arnold himself wrote to tell Joslin that, while his diabetes was not causing him any difficulty, the vision in his right eye was poor and his right shoulder stiff.[41] Joslin responded separately to each note, telling Mrs. Burns that control of Arnold's diabetes was the best possible tonic and suggesting to Arnold that X-ray therapy for bursitis of the shoulder, which had aided many other patients, might help. As always, Joslin also offered to see Arnold.[42]

Then, within a week, trouble turned into tragedy. Arnold explained in a neatly written letter to Root that he had recently switched jobs and was working in another garage.

> The second day there my right eye went blind so [that I can] only see light and dark. It was easier then to see with the left eye, [until] last Sunday [when] the left eye broke so I can hardly see news print. The garage people were afraid I'd get hurt so laid me off for a month to see if [my vision] will improve. . . . I called you last Monday afternoon but you were away. I called . . . [the ophthalmologist] and he said time was the only thing for the eye and advised no lifting or pulling.

I know you see people who if [they] stub their toe run to a doctor. I don't do that but what am I supposed to do? What can I expect? If I can't work how can I live? Please tell me what to do.[43]

At the end of this letter, just underneath Arnold's signature, were the initials "E. B.": his mother had transcribed the letter. Perhaps even Root—who had been on the front line of the battle against coma and was now embroiled in a new struggle to control the disease's delayed complications—began to feel a constricting, claustrophobic sensation as Arnold's world started to collapse around him.

Half a year later, Arnold spent a week in the Deaconess Hospital. He had a "hacking cough," and his ankles were greatly swollen. As the test results came back, the picture grew bleaker. His kidneys were now putting out massive amounts of albumin into the urine. An EKG of his heart showed that Arnold had had a silent heart attack, and now he was in a state of congestive heart failure. Root wrote to the young man's hometown doctor, "Arnold represents a typical case of the diabetic triopathy. I venture to enclose a reprint summarizing 155 of our patients who have this condition. . . . I see nothing for Arnold to do more than to carry on his diabetic treatment as carefully as possible."[44]

The article that Root referred to, published in 1954, framed the syndrome of diabetic triopathy (nerve, eye, and kidney damage) as both a clinical observation and a pointed therapeutic indictment. After showing that these complications often clustered together, Root and his coauthors argued that the eye and kidney problems were the result of poor diabetic control. They stratified their patients into four classes of diabetic control—excellent, good, fair, and poor—based upon criteria that incorporated medical parameters (for excellent control, "patient must never have been in coma") and measures of adherence to a strict diet and doctors' orders ("diet must have been weighed at least 80% of the time," daily urine tests "with a conscientious attempt to have the urine sugar free," and "regular physical examinations and laboratory tests"). The tacit moral of the paper was simple: those patients who had poor control ("medical advice neglected") suffered the consequences of higher rates of complications.[45] With this linkage of lax patient compliance to inadequate control and thence to complications, Arnold—once so proud of his independence from medical doctors and the restrictions of his disease—was in poor standing, medically and morally.

A month later, Arnold managed to write a note to Root, his handwriting frail and tremulous. He wanted to thank Root "for making the arrangements to get me in [to the hospital]. I want to thank you, Elliot Joslin, Priscilla White, and the others for the past service in getting the swelling out of my ankles and making it so I can lay down and get some sleep. And for keeping my expenses at a minimum."[46] The same day, Arnold started another letter to Root.

> Dear Howard Root, I have a few questions I would like to ask.
>
> 1. What is suppose to be wrong with me?
>
> 2. Why do I get out of breath when I try to do anything besides just sit around or walk slow? I used to be able to Work—Work hard anywhere from 8–16 hours a day. Now I am not good for 1/2 hours, feel like I am going to pass out.
>
> 3. They gave me some pills when I left the hospital. There were some big Red ones[,] the Bottle said to take 4 a day[,] the[y']re all gone, should I get more or not, don't feel any different with out them.
>
> 4. What did [you] think about my Left eye or do you think it will stay like it is or blow apart again? never mind this one [—] found out for my self—this is another day[,] got coughing last night[,] got up[,] lot of junk floating around in the left eye[,] have to keep moving my head around so I can see this page.
>
> 5. What makes my legs go numb when I sit or lay down?

Arnold concluded by stressing, "These are questions not complain[t]s. As I had 15 years w[h]ere I didn't have to take a back seat for any one[.] But since last Nov. I been riding under the back of a dump cart with all the other junk."[47]

Arnold was losing control not only over his health but over his conception of himself as independent, self-sustaining, and hard-working. A diabetic for as long as he probably could remember, who grew into adulthood proud of his ability to manage his ailment, he now confronted not only a grave medical condition but also an equally dire existential situation, as complications slowly eroded his self-image.[48] Root, who had anticipated this protracted deterioration,[49] wrote back to tell Arnold that he was "sorry to say that the trouble with you was the failure of your heart and . . . that means the heart muscle has lost some of its strength. Unfortunately, the diabetes spots in your eyes are the cause of the loss of vision." Then, in an avuncular way, Root tried to redirect Arnold's efforts toward coping. "I know it is very hard for you to take the back seat and take it slowly now, but I am afraid you will have to limit yourself in order to conserve the energy and protect yourself."[50]

In the middle of autumn three months later, 32-year-old Arnold wrote again: "My ankles have started to swell[;] they are about the size they were last spring. [T]he swelling goes part way up the legs and the legs are like two cakes of ice. I am starting to cough hard again and to cough in the night. I guess I sleep 2 or 3 hours a night. . . . I try not to be a pest with the questions. [B]ut if some thing happened, some people could say I didn't try to find out. . . . What do we do now?"[51]

By that winter, Arnold had suffered a stroke that paralyzed his right side. Two months later, he was hospitalized with a chief complaint of "Pain Right Leg." The leg was gangrenous, and so late that night, attempting to check his demise with a desperate intervention, the doctors amputated Arnold's leg at mid-thigh. The next morning the resident wrote, "Looks poorly—Cheyne Stokes respiration. [Then again, later that day] began to vomit coffee-ground material @ 6:30 pm. [Doctors] attempted to pass Levine Tube but [patient] appeared to aspirate vomitus and expired despite attempts to suction. Pronounced dead at 7:40 pm."[52] Arnold was 33 years old.

As was more customary then, Ethel permitted an autopsy, which reported "the major pathological findings":

> Healed infarcts of the myocardium.
> Mural thrombus of the left ventricle.
> Hypertrophy and dilatation of the left ventricle.
> Hypertrophy of the right ventricle.
> Dilatation of the pulmonary conus.
> Atherosclerosis of the coronary arteries.
> General arteriosclerosis.
> Recent infarct of the brain (left parietal lobe).
> Infarcts of the spleen and kidneys.
> Probable embolus in the right iliac artery.
> Right mid-thigh amputation.
> Bilateral pleural effusion, more marked at right.
> Collapse of the right lung.
> Marked congestion and edema of the left lung.
> Acute ulcers of the duodenum.
> Cholesterolosis of the gall bladder.
> Acute hemorrhagic cystitis.
> Slight edema of the left leg.
> Diabetes mellitus (clinical).

The cause of death, based on these findings, is due to respiratory failure.[53]

If the postmortem had probed beyond this litany of pathologies and sought out the human circumstances of this man who had been so ravaged by long-term diabetic complications, it might have produced a more concise and revealing report: the circumstances of Arnold's death, like his 29 years of prolonged diabetic life, had been shaped by medical intervention.

Shortly after Arnold's death, the operating surgeon wrote to Allen Joslin (Elliott's son, who had been the attending physician), "Just a note to tell you how sorry I am that we could not do more for your patient, Mr. Arnold Burns. I think the amputation that was done probably did get ahead of his gas gangrene but there were too many other problems to expect to get away with this in a man so sick. It is certainly a tragedy to see this condition in a patient who is so young."[54]

Allen Joslin sent condolences to Ethel, observing, "Arnold, was a most faithful patient as you know. . . . Your son did much better than all our diabetic children to date. We regret that some of our patients with over 30 years of insulin have complications. . . . His problems at the time of his passing were many."[55] Since Ethel had requested the autopsy findings, she also received a copy and an offer to answer any questions. A week later, she thanked Allen Joslin for the report, adding that she was "trying to straighten his financial affairs, I will be slow but will take care of them." Then, summing up not only the last letter she wrote to the clinic but, essentially, a whole dimension of Arnold's life, she went on to say: "I would like to take this time to thank all of the Joslin Clinic who were so kind to Arnold and also the nurses, Doctors, and all at the Deaconess, you know he called it his second home down there and felt it belonged to him."[56]

### The Want of Control

Looking back in 1954, Elliott Joslin recalled "the ideas of the leading apostles in diabetes in the last century," all of whom believed adamantly in the virtue of control and sought to achieve it through diet. Then "insulin arrived and diabetics lived rather than died. . . . Patients treated with insulin did so much better than ever before that a relaxation in the management of the disease seemed harmless." Joslin continued, his rhetorical tone rising, to note how "the warning statistics of doctors schooled in the treatment of diabetes were decried. . . . Against this background of apostasy, therefore, it is heartening now to read of the advocacy of control of the disease by those who have witnessed the results of the lack of it."[57]

For Joslin and other American practitioners throughout the 20th century, the central ambition of diabetic management—and its chief frustration—has been the want of control. The eagerness with which physicians have pursued this elusive objective, and in what directions, have distinguished various styles of managing the disease. Joslin may have declared partial victory at midcentury, but the advance of an alternative clinical style, which was less stringent regarding control and more concerned that patients live "normal" lives, would put his beliefs on the defensive for several decades. Since the 1950s, physicians have debated whether control could prevent long-term complications, and if so, how effectively. In 1993, the published results of a large clinical trial argued that Joslin was essentially right; patients placed on tight-control regimens, compared with those under normal diabetic care, lowered their risk of delayed complications markedly.[58] But this reduction of risk, important though it is, does not settle a more fundamental argument: even if the means of better diabetic control are now "at our door," the questions of what measures should we take to pursue control, and at what personal consequence to patients' lives, remain open, beyond the dictates of statistical data.

In many ways, what has compelled physicians to align themselves on one side or another of the control issue has never been a simple assessment of physiological efficacy but rather a complex set of ideas and ideals. The Joslin group structured their diabetic management around the ideal of seizing control of the disease, preventing all complications, and extending life at virtually any cost. Their collective commitment to this ideal of complete control was entrenched so deeply that it became a sacred ideal, beyond criticism, connected to other fundamental dichotomies, natural and moral:[59] control versus laxity; health versus sickness; life versus death; virtue versus sin. In one sense, Arnold owed his life to the uncompromising commitment that underwrote this scheme, as these values had propelled innovators such as Joslin forward as they pushed back the boundaries of what was medically possible, adding years to diabetic lives.

And yet, as Arnold's case illustrates so poignantly, these same values often imposed stern judgments and harsh trade-offs. When his complications first emerged, and then as his medical problems mounted, Arnold carried the burden not simply of his failing health but also of the medical attitudes that construed complications as the result of poor patient compliance and control—"medical advice neglected." Finally, near the end of Arnold's life, when gangrene was poised to cause his death, his doctors' aggressive interventions sacrificed his final hours in an uncompromising pursuit of medical control over death.

Arnold's experience encompassed all these paradoxes and dilemmas of medical practice and its connected ideals. Viewed from this perspective, his experience with diabetes transcends the inexorable course of an aberrant metabolism, becoming a powerful commentary on the often contradictory aims built into modern medicine. Arnold's case exhibits the bittersweet irony of an illness transformed by a therapeutic style of relentless control, tracing the mortal arc from a life saved, from the moment of clinical salvation through to the end of that life. What medicine had given to Arnold, it had—in an untoward alliance with the disease—taken away.

The twists and turns in this latter-day morality play remind us that the complex world of therapeutic options and decisions rarely admits to perfect solutions. Instead, clinicians and patients have long struggled with the inescapable trade-offs posed when limited knowledge and capacity to heal confront human disease and mortality. The choices that these players have made reflected the circumstances and temper of their times as well as idiosyncratic preference. Joslin embodied an ethos widely prevalent in 20th-century American medicine and society: the desire to control disease and death. His achievements as both architect and spokesman for intensive diabetic management paralleled treatment strategies developed by other physicians in other specialties, evident from intensive care units to high-risk obstetrical practices to trauma surgical services. These endeavors express values that patients and physicians alike have promulgated, almost to the point where medical control has become a fetish, to be viewed as selfless or high-minded or even self-protective, providing some assurance in the face of capricious and seemingly cruel diseases.[60] And, no doubt, the exhaustive attention and increasingly sophisticated interventions of this therapeutic approach have benefited many patients, diabetic and otherwise, and will continue to do so in the future as more diseases are transmuted from acute to chronic forms.

From this point of view, the story of Arnold, his mother, Ethel, and the doctors who treated him emphasizes the central role that ideals of controlling disease have played in shaping patient care. Joslin, who combined remarkable dedication and integrity in his quest for a better diabetic world, was but one physician who espoused such ideals—ideals that together with brave new ideas and innovations have forged the predominant style of modern American medical therapeutics.

## Notes

The original article has been abridged for this edition.

1  Intake sheet, 22 March 1927; and, on back of intake sheet, past medical history in Priscilla White's handwriting; both in the Joslin Diabetes Center Historical Archive (JDCA), Boston, Massachusetts.

2  Elliott P. Joslin (EPJ) to local medical doctor (LMD), 29 March 1927, JDCA.

3  Ibid., 14 April 1927.

4  Hudson, in *Disease and Its Control*, has examined past attempts to control disease as mediated (in the broadest sense) by understanding disease either ontologically or physiologically. This chapter operates within a different analytic framework, as it tries to understand more explicitly the connections among ideas of disease, therapeutic ideals, and actual patient care. Robert P. Hudson, *Disease and Its Control: The Shaping of Modern Thought* (Westport, Conn.: Greenwood Press, 1983). Two major studies of therapeutics that have considered aspects of these relationships are Erwin H. Ackerknecht, *Therapeutics from the Primitives to the 20th Century. With an Appendix: History of Dietetics* (New York: Hafner Press, 1973); and John Harley Warner, *The Therapeutic Perspective: Medical Practice, Knowledge, and Identity in America, 1820–1885* (Cambridge, Mass.: Harvard University Press, 1986).

5  A similar tale has been told of renal dialysis and organ transplantation by Renée C. Fox and Judith P. Swazey, *The Courage to Fail: A Social View of Organ Transplants and Dialysis*, 2nd ed. (Chicago: University of Chicago Press, 1978).

6  Michael Bliss, *The Discovery of Insulin* (Chicago: University of Chicago Press, 1982); Joseph H. Barach, "Historical Facts in Diabetes," *Annals of Medical History* 10 (1928): 387–401; Martin M. Nothman, "The History of the Discovery of Pancreatic Diabetes," *Bulletin of the History of Medicine* 28 (1954): 272–274. This genealogy of the theory was put forward by just about every contemporary physician that commented on the discovery of insulin, including Joslin.

7  Elliott P. Joslin, "The Changing Diabetic Clientele," *Transactions of the Association of American Physicians* 39 (1924): 304–307, 304. Only Banting and Macleod were awarded the prize, which served to further inflame the credit dispute within the group (Bliss, *Discovery of Insulin*). Michael Bliss has recently reevaluated Best's role in the discovery and development of insulin in "Rewriting Medical History: Charles Best and the Banting and Best Myth," *Journal of the History of Medicine and Allied Sciences* 48 (1993): 253–274.

8  Joslin continued his line of thinking further in his article "Routine Treatment of Diabetes with Insulin," *Journal of the American Medical Association* 80 (1923): 1581–83, 1581: "Insulin does not allow a diabetic to eat anything he desires . . . It is true that heretofore there has never been anything discovered as valuable for the diabetic as insulin; but diabetes, though subdued, is not yet conquered."

9  The sense in which insulin "conquered" diabetes—and how clinicians thought about the impact of this dramatic but noncurative treatment—is strikingly analogous to the "con-

quest" of pernicious anemia through the use of the liver extract therapy developed by Minot and Murphy; see Keith Wailoo, *Drawing Blood: Technology and Disease Identity in Twentieth-Century America* (Baltimore: Johns Hopkins University Press, 1997). Analogous thoughts and behaviors can also be found regarding not just other potent biological compounds but also remarkable technological innovation such as renal dialysis and organ transplant; see Fox and Swazey, *Courage to Fail*.

10  My understanding of Dr. Priscilla White was deepened by her colleague, M. Donna Younger; the quotation regarding ice cream is from an interview that I conducted with Dr. Younger on 1 July 1992 at the Joslin Diabetes Center. I have also been guided by White's personal papers, which contain many heartfelt letters from patients; these are housed in the Schlesinger Library on the History of Women in America, Radcliffe College, Cambridge, Mass. For a glimpse at White's extensive work on diabetic pregnancy, see "Diabetes Mellitus in Pregnancy," *Clinics in Perinatology* 1 (1974): 331–347.

11  EPJ to Ethel Burns (EB), 17 April 1928, JDCA.

12  EB to EPJ, 22 November 1930, JDCA.

13  EPJ to EB, 24 November 1930, JDCA.

14  In 1934, a social worker estimated that the weekly cost of insulin and other routine materials was $1.75. Genevieve Peterson, "The Social Aspects of Diabetes: A Study of Sixty Cases," *New England Journal of Medicine* 211 (1934): 397–402. In 1947, Joslin reported that the average diabetic hospitalization cost totaled $269; see "Cost of Hospital Care [unsigned editorial]," *New England Journal of Medicine* 237 (1947): 461–462.

15  EB to EPJ, 8 February 1929, JDCA.

16  Ibid., 9 February 1932.

17  Outpatient chart, 30 March 1933, JDCA.

18  EB to EPJ, 12 April 1933, JDCA.

19  Joslin, "Cost of Hospital Care"; numerous letters to patients and doctors contained in other medical records document his waiving of fees.

20  Joslin, "Abolishing Diabetic Coma," *Journal of the American Medical Association* 93 (1929): 33; and "Diabetic Coma [unsigned editorial]," *New England Journal of Medicine* 201 (1929): 1007–8, 1007.

21  One record from the JDCA indicates that a young man had first come to Joslin in 1926, having "two days ago omitted insulin because he was out of insulin and alcohol . . . Does not know how to test urine." Later, he died after lapsing into coma in his hometown hospital, where (according to LMD) "insolin [*sic*] and glucose injections were of no avail." Reports of such events were not uncommon in the charts I have examined.

22  Inpatient medical chart, 7 July 1934, JDCA. Arnold was admitted in coma with a blood sugar of 0.68 percent (that is, 680 milligrams/deciliter [mg/dl] of blood) and blood carbon dioxide of 11 volumes percent. He was treated with 750 cc of intravenous normal saline, a 1,500 cc clysis, and insulin, as follows: 20 units every half hour from 6:40 P.M. until 9:10 P.M., then 40 units at 9:25 P.M. and 9:50 P.M. His blood sugar at 10 P.M. was 0.19 percent; at 5 A.M., 0.04; he was given 5 grams of glucose intravenously for a reaction at 6:30 A.M.; he then stabilized.

23  Priscilla White (PW) to EB, 16 July 1934, JDCA.

24  Although this fact is beyond the scope of this chapter, I should note that from the particular crisis of coma, Joslin and his colleague extended the operational paradigm of intensive

control to other diabetic problems, such as pregnancy, then to the treatment of infections (especially after the advent of antibiotics), and more broadly to the daily management of a patient's regimen of diet, exercise, and insulin.

25 R. T. Woodyatt to Elmer L. Sevringhaus, 26 December 1929, Sevringhaus Papers, American Philosophical Society Library, Philadelphia, Pa.

26 For a summary of these diets, which along with those of Newburgh and Marsh, permitted much more fat than had become customary, see Rollin T. Woodyatt, "Objects and Methods of Diet Adjustment in Diabetes," *Transactions of the Association of American Physicians* 36 (1921): 269–92.

27 R. T. Woodyatt to Elmer L. Sevringhaus, 26 December 1929, Sevringhaus Papers, American Philosophical Society Library, Philadelphia, Pa. The portrait of Rollin Turner Woodyatt (1878–1953) is based upon materials in the Woodyatt obituary file (including a typescript copy of the 21 December 1953 eulogy delivered by Arthur R. Colwell), which is held in the Faculty Members Biographical Files, 1837–1942, at the Rush-Presbyterian-St. Luke's Medical Center Archives, Chicago, Ill.

28 The position outlined by Woodyatt, in both its scientific reasoning and its assessment of "the good life," was held by many physicians. The controversy over the need for "tight" control raged from the 1940s onward, with Edward Tolstoi often championing a deemphasis of glycosuria; see Edward Tolstoi, "Treatment of Diabetes Mellitus: The Controversy of the Past Decade," *Cincinnati Journal of Medicine* 30 (1949): 1–7.

29 This point, in a different context, is made by Warner, *Therapeutic Perspective.*

30 EB to PW, 5 May 1938, JDCA.

31 PW to EB, 9 May 1938, JDCA.

32 EB to PW, 27 May 1938, JDCA. These hypoglycemic reactions were precisely what Woodyatt, in his therapeutic strategy outlined above, wanted to avoid.

33 This vigorous image of success was literally the "portrait" presented in the frontispiece of Joslin's 1928 textbook (which displayed a photograph of a twenty-year-old woman, ten years after her diagnosis of diabetes, grasping a tennis racquet). Joslin continued to project similar images of vitality throughout his publications, culminating in the numerous photographs contained in his 1956 manual. In a similar vein, but without the visual rhetoric, Priscilla White presented statistical data regarding various measures of "achievement" of her juvenile patients; see Priscilla White, "Natural Course and Prognosis of Juvenile Diabetes," *Diabetes* 5 (November 1956): 445–450.

34 "Of What Shall Diabetics Die?" [unsigned editorial], *New England Journal of Medicine* 210 (1934): 43.

35 Paul Kimmelstiel and Clifford Wilson, "Intercapillary Lesions in the Glomeruli of the Kidney," *American Journal Pathology* 12 (1936): 83–98.

36 White, "Natural Course."

37 Arnold Burns (AB) to EPJ, 30 March 1948, JDCA.

38 EB to EPJ, 1 October 1949, JDCA.

39 Howard F. Root (HFR) to AB, 17 November 1951, JDCA. Root reported to Arnold the following clinical information: a blood pressure of 140/78 mg Hg; fasting blood sugar 85 mg/dl; nonprotein nitrogen 32 mg/dl; urine sugar 5.5 percent (that is, 5.5 mg/dl), urine albumin 20 mg percent (that is, 20 mg/dl); X-ray examinations normal; and Grade 4 diabetic retinitis.

40 EB to EPJ, 10 March 1954, JDCA.

41  AB to EPJ, 15 March 1954, JDCA.

42  EPJ to EB, 16 March 1954, and EPJ to AB, 18 March 1954, JDCA.

43  AB to HFR, 7 November 1954, JDCA.

44  Inpatient medical chart, 28 April 1955, and HFR to LMD, 10 May 1955, JDCA.

45  Howard F. Root, William H. Pote, and Hans Frehner, "Triopathy of Diabetes: Sequence of Neuropathy, Retinopathy, and Nephropathy in One Hundred Fifty-Five Patients," *Archives of Internal Medicine* 94 (1954): 931–941.

46  AB to HFR, 13 June 1955, JDCA.

47  Ibid.

48  Renée C. Fox's study of critically ill patients, conducted during the early 1950s, identified similar problems and methods of coping; see *Experiment Perilous: Physicians and Patients Facing the Unknown* (1959; reprint, Philadelphia: University of Pennsylvania Press, 1974).

49  HFR to local cardiologist, 10 May 1955, JDCA.

50  HFR to AB, 16 June 1955, JDCA.

51  AB to HFR, 16 October 1955, JDCA.

52  Inpatient medical chart, 25 March 1956, JDCA. Cheyne-Stokes respirations are a gravely disturbed breathing pattern, while "coffee-ground vomit" indicates gastrointestinal bleeding; a Levine tube would be passed through the mouth to the stomach in an attempt to control the bleeding.

53  William A. Meissner, M.D. [pathologist], to EPJ, 28 March 1956, JDCA.

54  Frank C. Wheelock Jr. [operating surgeon who collaborated with McKittrick in surgical practice] to Allen Joslin, 3 April 1956, JDCA. These comments can be viewed as expressing and maintaining a surgical community's values and ethical positions, similar to those explored by Charles L. Bosk in *Forgive and Remember: Managing Medical Failure* (Chicago: University of Chicago Press, 1979).

55  Allen Joslin to EB, 2 April 1956, JDCA.

56  EB to Allen Joslin, 11 April 1956, JDCA.

57  Elliott P. Joslin, "A Renaissance of the Control of Diabetes [guest editorial]," *Journal of the American Medical Association* 156 (1954): 1584–85. The most blasphemous document, from Joslin's point of view, probably would have been Edward Tolstoi's *Living with Diabetes*, a book published in 1952 expressly for the lay diabetic audience, preaching looser glycemic control in order to promote a more "normal" lifestyle. *Living with Diabetes* (New York: Crown, 1952). For both sides of the control argument, see the editorials by George M. Joslin, "'Free Diet' for Diabetes, Pro [editorial]," *Diabetes* 1 (1952): 487–488; and Alexander Marble, "'Free Diet' for Diabetes, Con [editorial]," *Diabetes* 1 (1952): 488–489.

58  The Diabetes Control and Complications Trial Research Group, "The Effects of Intensive Treatment of Diabetes on the Development and Progression of Long-Term Complications in Insulin-Dependent Diabetes Mellitus," *New England Journal of Medicine* 329 (1993): 977–986.

59  This argument draws on the work of Mary Douglas, summarized in *How Institutions Think* (Syracuse, N.Y.: Syracuse University Press, 1986).

60  For a discussion of these issues, see Renée C. Fox, "The Human Condition of Health Professionals," in *Essays in Medical Sociology: Journey into the Field*, 2nd ed., rev. and enl. (New Brunswick, N.J.: Transaction Books, 1988).

## Spence + Lila
Bobbie Ann Mason

### One

On the way to the hospital in Paducah, Spence notices the row of signs along the highway: WHERE WILL YOU BE IN ETERNITY? Each word is on a white cross. The message reminds him of the old Burma-Shave signs. His wife, Lila, beside him, has been quiet during the trip, which takes forty minutes in his Rabbit. He didn't take her car because it has a hole in the muffler, but she has complained about his car ever since he cut the seat belts off to deactivate the annoying warning buzzer.

As they pass the Lone Oak shopping center, on the outskirts of Paducah, Lila says fretfully, "I don't know if the girls will get here."

"They're supposed to be here by night," Spence reminds her. Ahead, a gas station marquee advertises a free case of Coke with a tune-up.

Catherine, their younger daughter, has gone to pick up Nancy at the airport in Nashville. Although Lila objected to the trouble and expense, Nancy is flying all the way from Boston. Cat lives nearby, and Nancy will stay with her. Nancy offered to stay with Spence, so he wouldn't be alone, but he insisted he would be all right.

When Cat brought Lila home from the doctor the day before and Lila said, "They think it's cancer," the words ran through him like electricity. She didn't cry all evening, and when he tried to hold her, he couldn't speak. They sat in the living room in their recliner chairs, silent and scared, watching TV just as they usually did. Before she sat down for the evening, she worked busily in the kitchen, freezing vegetables from the garden and cooking food for him to eat during her stay in the hospital. He

Bobbie Ann Mason, Selections from *Spence + Lila.* © 1988 by Bobbie Ann Mason. Reprinted by permission of HarperCollins Publishers, Inc.

couldn't eat any supper except a bowl of cereal, and she picked at some ham and green beans.

He knew she had not been feeling well for months; she'd had dizzy spells and she had lost weight. The doctor at the local clinic told her to come back in three months if she kept losing weight, but Cat insisted on taking her mother to Paducah. The doctors were better there, Cat insisted, in that know-it-all manner both his daughters had. Cat, who was careless with money, didn't even think to ask what the specialists would charge. When she brought Lila home, it was late—feeding time. Spence was at the pond feeding the ducks, with Oscar, the dog. When Oscar saw the car turn into the driveway, he tore through the soybean field toward the house, as if he, too, were anxious for a verdict.

They had told Lila that her dizzy spells were tiny strokes. They also found a knot in her right breast. They wanted to take the knot out and do a test on it, and if it was cancer they would take her whole breast off, right then. It was an emergency, Lila explained. They couldn't deal with the strokes until they got the knot out. Spence imagined the knot growing so fast it would eat her breast up if she waited another day or two.

They're crawling through the traffic on the edge of Paducah. When he was younger, Spence used to come and watch the barges on the river. They glided by confidently, like miniature flattops putting out to sea. He has wanted to take Lila for a cruise on the *Delta Queen*, the luxury steamboat that paddles all the way to New Orleans, but he hasn't been able to bring himself to do it.

He turns on the radio and a Rod Stewart song blares out.

"Turn that thing off!" Lila yells.

"I thought you needed a little entertainment," he says, turning the sound down.

She rummages in her purse for a cigarette, her third on the trip. "They won't let me have any cigarettes tonight, so I better smoke while I got a chance."

"I'll take them things and throw 'em away," he says.

"You better not."

She cracks the window open at the top to let the smoke out. Her face is the color of cigarette ashes. She looks bad.

"I guess it's really cancer," she says, blowing out smoke. "The X-ray man said it was cancer."

"How would he know? He ain't even a doctor."

"He's seen so many, he would know."

"He ain't paid to draw that conclusion," Spence says. "Why did he want to scare you like that? Didn't the doctor say he'd have to wait till they take the knot out and look at it?"

"Yeah, but—" She fidgets with her purse, wadding her cigarette package back into one of the zipper pockets. "The X-ray man sees those X-rays all day long. He knows more about X-rays than a doctor does."

Spence turns into the hospital parking lot, unsure where to go. The eight-story hospital cuts through the humid, hazy sky, like a stray sprig of milo growing up in a bean field. A car pulls out in front of him. Spence's reactions are slow today, but he hits the brakes in time.

"I think I'll feel safer in the hospital," Lila says.

Walking from the parking lot, he carries the small bag she packed. He suspects there is a carton of cigarettes in it. Cat keeps trying to get Lila to quit, but Lila has no willpower. Once Cat gave her a cassette tape on how to quit smoking, but Lila accidentally ran it through the washing machine. It was in a shirt pocket. "Accidentally on purpose," Cat accused her. Cat even told Lila once that cigarettes caused breast cancer. But Spence believes worry causes it. She worries about Cat, the way she has been running around with men she hardly knows since her divorce last year. It's a bad example for her two small children, and Lila is afraid the men aren't serious about Cat. Lila keeps saying no one will want to marry a woman with two extra mouths to feed.

Now Lila says, "I want you to supervise that garden. The girls won't know how to take care of it. That corn needs to be froze, and the beans are still coming in."

"Don't worry about your old garden," he says impatiently. "Maybe I'll mow it down."

"Spence!" Lila cries, grabbing his arm tightly. "Don't you go and mow down my garden!"

"You work too hard on it," he says. "We don't need all that grub anymore for just us two."

"The beans is about to begin a second round of blooming," she says. "I want to let most of them make into shellies and save some for seed. And I don't want the corn to get too old."

The huge glass doors of the hospital swing open, and a nurse pushes out an old woman in a wheelchair. The woman is bony and pale, with a cluster of kinfolks in bluejeans around her. Her aged hands, folded in her lap, are spotted like little bird dogs. The air-conditioning blasts Spence and Lila as they enter, and he feels as though they are walking into a meat locker.

## Two

She felt that lump weeks ago, but she didn't mention it then. When she and Spence returned from a trip to Florida recently, she told Cat about it, and Cat started pestering her to see a specialist. The knot did feel unusual, like a piece of gristle. The magazines said you would know it was different. Lila never examined her breasts the way they said to do, because her breasts were always full of lumps anyway—from mastitis, which she had several times. Her breasts are so enormous she cannot expect to find a little knot. Spence says her breasts are like cow bags. He has funny names for them, like the affectionate names he had for his cows when they used to keep milk cows. Names like Daisy and Bossy. Petunia. Primrose. It will be harder on him if she loses one of her breasts than it will be on her. Women can stand so much more than men can.

She makes him leave the hospital early, wanting to be alone so she can smoke a cigarette in peace. After he brought her in, he paced around, then went downstairs for a Coke. Now he leaves to go home, and she watches him from behind as he trudges down the corridor, hugging himself in the cold. Lila is glad she brought her housecoat, but even with it she is afraid she will take pneumonia.

In the lounge, she smokes and plays with a picture puzzle laid out on a card table. Someone has pieced most of the red barn and pasture, and a vast blue sky remains to be done. Lila loves puzzles. When she was little, growing up at her uncle's, she had a puzzle of a lake scene with a castle. She worked that puzzle until the design was almost worn away. The older folks always kidded her, but she kept working the puzzle devotedly. She always loved the satisfying snap of two pieces going together. It was like knowing something for sure.

Her son Lee towers in the doorway of the lounge. She stands up, surprised.

"Did you get off work early?" He works at Ingersoll-Rand.

"No. I just took off an hour, and I have to go back and work till nine. They're working me overtime this month." He has lines on his face and he is only thirty-two.

He hugs her silently. He's so tall her head pokes his armpit, where he has always been ticklish.

"I didn't know you were that sick in Florida," he says. "We shouldn't have dragged you through Disney World."

"I knew something was wrong, but I didn't know what." She explains

63

the details of the X-rays and the operation, then says, "I'm going to lose my breast, Lee."

"You are?" The lines on his face freeze. He needs a shave.

"They won't know till they get in there, but if it's cancer they'll go ahead and take it out."

"Which one?"

"This one," she says, cupping her right breast.

A woman with frizzy red hair hobbles into the lounge, her hospital gown exposing her fat, doughy knees. "I was looking for my husband," she says, "but I reckon he ain't here."

Lila waits for the woman to leave, then laughs. She's still holding her breast. "You don't remember sucking on these, do you, Lee?" She loves to tease her son. "You sucked me dry and I had to put you on a bottle after two months. I couldn't make enough milk to feed you."

With an embarrassed grin, Lee looks out the window. "I believe you're making that up."


**Four**

Lila says, "They sure don't let you get lonesome here—all the traipsing in and out they do at all hours."

Cat and Nancy are hovering over the bed, staring at her with an unnatural sort of eagerness. "Did you sleep?" Cat asks.

"Off and on," says Lila. She tries to sit up against the pillow, but she feels woozy from this morning's medicine. "That coffee last night made me jumpy, but they give me some pills and a shot."

Nancy says, "That's outrageous! There was no good reason to give you coffee. You should have refused it."

Cat's earrings dangle in Lila's face. Lila's mind feels fuzzy, far away. She is afraid the operating room will be cold.

"Are you scared?" Nancy asks, holding Lila's hand.

"They work you over too much for you to be scared. I haven't had time to think." Lila squeezes Nancy's hand and reaches for Cat's. "You girls are being good to me," she says. "I sure am lucky."

"Well, we care about you," Cat says.

"You're going to be just fine, Mom," says Nancy. "You're tough."

"I guess I better say goodbye to my jug," Lila says, laughing and looking down at herself. "If Spence don't hurry on here, he's going to miss his chance."

Just then Spence appears, still in short sleeves. Yesterday she tried to tell him to wear long sleeves, but he wouldn't listen to her. After giving Nancy a hug, he steps back and eyes her up and down to see how much older she seems.

"You look poor as a snake," he says. "Why didn't you bring Robert?"

"He's going off to camp tomorrow. Jack's taking him up to New Hampshire. It's the same place he went last year, where they go on treks into the mountains."

"Bring him down here. I'll see that he communes with nature." Spence grins at Nancy.

"I'm sure you will. You'll have him out planting soybeans." Nancy twists out of a nurse's way.

"It would be good for him," Lila says sleepily. "Working out in the fields would teach him something."

She closes her eyes, vaguely listening to Spence and the girls talk. If this is her time to go, she should be ready. And she has her family with her, except for Lee, who had to work. She feels she is looking over her whole life, holding it up to see how it has turned out—like a piece of sewing. She can see Cat trying on a dress Lila has made for her, and Lila checks to see whether it needs taking up. She turns up the hem, jerks the top to see how it fits across the shoulders, considers an extra tuck in the waist. In a recurrent dream she has had for years, she is trying to finish a garment, sewing fast against the clock.

They are still chattering nervously around her when the surgeon appears. He's young, with sensitive hands that look skilled at delicate finger work. Lila always notices people's fingers. Nancy and Cat keep asking questions, but Lila is sleepy and can't follow all that he is saying. Then he moves closer to her and says, "If the biopsy shows a malignancy, I'm going to recommend a modified radical mastectomy. I'll remove the breast tissue and the lymph nodes under the arm. But I'll leave the chest muscles. If you follow the physical therapy, then you'll have full use of your arm and you'll be just fine." He smiles reassuringly. He resembles a cousin of Lila's—Whip Stanton, a little man with a lisp and a wife with palsy.

"How small would the lump have to be for you to recommend a lumpectomy instead?" Nancy asks the doctor.

"Infinitesimal," he says. "It's better to get it all out and be sure. This way is more certain."

"Well, more and more doctors are recommending lumpectomies instead of mastectomies," Nancy argues. "What I'm asking is, what is the dividing line? How large should the lump be for the mastectomy to be preferable?"

Lila sees Spence cringe. Nancy has always asked questions and done things differently, just to be contrary. "Nancy, Nancy, quite contrary," they used to tease her.

The doctor shrugs and leans against the wall. "It depends on a number of factors," he says. "You can't reduce it to a question of size. If it's an aggressive tumor, a fast-growing one, then a smaller lump might be more dangerous than one that has grown slowly over a longer period of time. And my suspicion is that this is an aggressive tumor. You can get a second opinion if you want to, but we've got her prepped, and if the second opinion was in favor of a lumpectomy, then wouldn't you have to go for a third opinion, so you could take two out of three? But in this case, time is of the essence." The doctor grins at Lila. "What do you think, Mrs. Culpepper? You look like a pretty smart lady."

"Why, you're just a little whippersnapper," Lila says. "All the big words make me bumfuzzled. I guess you know your stuff, but I got you beat when it comes to producing pretty daughters." She has heard he is single, and she heard the nurses joking with him. She can't keep her mind on the conversation. It's as though she's floating around the room, dipping in and out of the situation, the way the nurses do.

**Eight**

Lila feels as though she has been left out in a field for the buzzards. The nurses are in at all hours, making no special effort to be quiet—a nurse who checks dressings, another one who changes dressings, a nurse with blood-thinner shots three times a day, a nurse with breathing-machine treatments, various nurses' aides who check temperature and blood pressure, the cleaning woman, the mail lady, the priest and nuns from the hospital, the girls who fill the water jugs, the woman who brings the meal trays, the candy stripers selling toiletries and candy and magazines from a cart. Lila can't keep track of all the nurses who come to check her drainage tube—squirting the murky fluid out of the plastic collection bottle, measuring the fluid intake and output, writing on charts. The nurses walk her around the entire third floor twice a day, accompanied by her i.v. bag, wheeling on a stand. Spence is nervous, bursting in anxiously, unable to stick around. And the girls are in and out, bringing her little things—a basket of flowers from the gift shop downstairs and some perfume. Lee and Joy brought a rose in a milk-glass bud vase. The church sent pink daisies. The old woman in the other bed has no flowers.

The surgeon told Lila she could live without a breast. "You couldn't live without a head, or a liver, or a heart," he said when he informed her in the recovery room that he had removed her breast. "But you can live without a breast. You'll be surprised."

"It would be like living without balls," Lila replied. "You'd find that surprising too, but you could probably get along without them."

Lila is not sure she said that aloud, and remembering it now, she is embarrassed that she might have, under the influence of the drugs. She's surprised Nancy hasn't said the same thing to the doctor's face.

Lila hears the old woman in the other bed grunting and complaining. "I'll not leave here alive!" she shouted when a nurse gave her a bath. "You're wasting your time fooling with me."

By the second day after her surgery, Lila is no longer hooked to the i.v. She plucks at the hospital gown in front where her bandage itches. The drainage tubes irritate her skin. She feels weak, but restless. "I'm afraid my blood's too thin already," she tells the nurse who comes with the blood-thinner shot.

"No, this is what the doctor wanted," the nurse says.

"I'm getting poked so full of holes I'm like a sifter bottom."

Besides the shots, there are the tests. They have wheeled her into the cold basement three times to run her through their machines. They have scanned her bones, her liver, her whole body, looking for loose cancer cells. Now the cancer doctor comes in to tell Lila the results of the tests: The cancer has spread to two out of the seventeen lymph nodes that were removed. Spence isn't there yet, but Cat and Nancy fire questions at him. Lila's head spins as the doctor explains that once the cancer has reached the lymph nodes, it has gone into the bloodstream, and then it can end up anywhere. The news doesn't quite register.

"I'm recommending chemotherapy," the doctor says.

"Is that cobalt?" Lila asks weakly. The doctor is young and reminds her of the odd-looking preacher who led the revival at church last year. The preacher had a long nose and wore a gold shiny suit.

The doctor says, "No. This will be a combination of three drugs— Cytoxan, methotrexate and 5FU." He explains that she will have a chart showing two weeks of treatments, then a three-week rest period, then two weeks of treatments, and so on. She will get both pills and shots. Like dogs teaming up on a rabbit, Cat and Nancy jump on him about side effects.

"This particular treatment is tolerated very well," he says. "That's not to say there won't be side effects. A little hair loss, a little nausea. Some people react more adversely than others."

Lila can't keep her mind on what he's saying. "I've got plenty of hair," she says, tugging at her curls. "And it's coarse, like horse hair." The last permanent she got didn't take on top.

"You're going to have to lay off the smoking too," the doctor says, consulting his clipboard.

"They won't let me smoke here," Lila says. She bummed a cigarette from a visitor in the lounge the night before, but it burned her lungs and tasted bitter. She couldn't finish it.

The cancer doctor says now, "Cigarettes will interfere with the chemotherapy."

"See!" Nancy says triumphantly. "Doctor's orders. And you wouldn't listen to us."

"These girls snitched my cigarettes," Lila says to the doctor. "Is that any way to treat an old woman that's stove up in the hospital?"

"Best thing for you," the doctor says with a slight grin.


**Fourteen**

A woman from the mastectomy support group arrives the next afternoon, bringing Lila a temporary pad to stuff in her brassiere until she can be measured for a permanent one. Lila feels embarrassed because both her daughters and Spence are right there. Spence is reading the newspaper noisily, rattling the pages and jerking them out smooth. Lila worries about his nerves.

"It's called a prosthesis," the woman explains. Lila did not catch her name. Cheerful and little, pert as a wren, she stands beside the bed, speaking to Lila like a school-teacher. She presents Lila with the object, which is in a plastic bag.

"Law," says Lila. "That weighs a ton." It reminds her of those sandbags used to hold down temporary signs on the highway.

"I can tell you're surprised," the woman chirps. "We don't realize the weight we're carrying around. You can put a strain on your back if you don't get properly fitted. So don't just stuff your bra with any old thing to make it look right. It's got to feel right and it's got to be the right weight, or you can run into serious problems."

The woman says she has had a mastectomy herself, and presumably she is wearing one of these sandbags in her brassiere. Lila notices Spence squirming. Nancy and Cat don't jump on this woman the way they did on the doctors. Cat is playing solitaire and Nancy is reading a book. Mrs. Wright is asleep.

The woman tells a long tale about her own mastectomy. "I was worried about recurrence," she says. "And I did have a lump to come in the other breast. It was tested and it was benign, but I made the decision to have the second breast removed too. I just didn't want to take the chance of having cancer again. Now that may sound extreme to you, but it was just the way I felt. So I'm free from worry, and the prosthesis works just fine."

The woman's little points are as perky as her personality. If the originals were that small, she probably doesn't miss them, Lila thinks. The woman talks awhile about balance, and then she talks about understanding. She has a packet of materials for Lila to read. "You may get depressed over losing part of your femininity," she says. "And we want you to know we're available to help." Lila listens carefully, but she can't think of anything to say.

"The doctors were skeptical when we started our organization," the woman says, leaning toward Lila and speaking in a confidential half-whisper. "But after we advertised, we had fifty women come to the first meeting. There was a great need for this, and we want you to know that we're there to serve you."

"Would I have to come all the way to Paducah?"

"Yes. That's where we hold our meetings, on the first Monday night of each month."

"Well, I don't get out much at night. And I don't like to drive on that Paducah highway."

"Let me urge you just to try it and see what it does for you. I'll give you the names of some people to contact." She talks on and on, about how the family should be understanding. In the packet are letters to daughters and sons and husbands. Spence and the girls are pretending they aren't there. "The letters say things that you may be uncomfortable saying, things you might be afraid to say, but they will explain your feelings at this delicate time when you need emotional support. All you have to do is send the appropriate letter to your daughters and your husband and to your sons, if you have any. It will be a nice surprise for them if you just send them in the mail. It's a much easier way for you to communicate your feelings."

"My girls have stood by me," Lila says, nodding proudly at Cat and Nancy. "And my boy works long hours and can't come as often, but he does when he can. Nancy flew all the way down here from New York."

"Boston," Nancy says, peering over her reading glasses.

"That's the same thing to us down here," the woman says with an apologetic smile.

"How much will this thing cost?" Lila asks. "If you charge by the pound, it might be high." She laughs at herself. She wonders why the woman didn't replace her breasts with big ones. Small-breasted women were always envious of Lila.

"The important thing is to get the proper fitting. With your fitting, and the bra and the prosthesis, the package comes to about a hundred and fifty dollars."

"Good night!" Lila and Spence cry simultaneously.

"But it's an important investment."

After the woman has gone, Spence says, "Will Medicare cover that?"

"I doubt it," Lila says. "I failed to ask her. Law, I hope I don't have to have false teeth anytime soon! I won't be able to keep track of that much stuff."

"You don't need that thing. We can rig you up something."

"Why, shoot, yes," Lila says. "I ain't spending a hundred and fifty dollars for a falsie."

Nancy laughs. "I read about a woman who stuffed her bra with buckshot, and she got stopped at the airport by the metal detector."

Cat says, "I heard about a woman who had an inflatable bra, and she went up in an airplane, and with the change in air pressure they exploded!"

They're all laughing, and Lila spontaneously tosses the prosthesis to Spence. "Catch!" she cries. Spence snatches it out of the air and flings it to Nancy and Nancy tosses it to Cat. Cat starts to throw it to Lila but stops herself, probably realizing Lila's right arm is weak. Lila is laughing so much her stitches hurt. Cat hands her the little sandbag and Lila says, "Well, it'll make a good pincushion."

They all laugh even harder then because Lila is in the habit of keeping stray straight pins and safety pins fastened to her blouse, and more than once in her life she has accidentally jabbed her breast with a pin.

## Silver Water
Amy Bloom

My sister's voice was like mountain water in a silver pitcher; the clear blue beauty of it cools you and lifts you up beyond your heat, beyond your body. After we went to see *La Traviata*, when she was fourteen and I was twelve, she elbowed me in the parking lot and said, "Check this out." And she opened her mouth unnaturally wide and her voice came out, so crystalline and bright that all the departing operagoers stood frozen by their cars, unable to take out their keys or open their doors until she had finished, and then they cheered like hell.

That's what I like to remember, and that's the story I told to all of her therapists. I wanted them to know her, to know that who they saw was not all there was to see. That before her constant tinkling of commercials and fast-food jingles there had been Puccini and Mozart and hymns so sweet and mighty you expected Jesus to come down off his cross and clap. That before there was a mountain of Thorazined fat, swaying down the halls in nylon maternity tops and sweatpants, there had been the prettiest girl in Arrandale Elementary School, the belle of Landmark Junior High. Maybe there were other pretty girls, but I didn't see them. To me, Rose, my beautiful blond defender, my guide to Tampax and my mother's moods, was perfect.

She had her first psychotic break when she was fifteen. She had been coming home moody and tearful, then quietly beaming, then she stopped coming home. She would go out into the woods behind our house and not come in until my mother went after her at dusk, and stepped gently into the briars and saplings and pulled her out, blank-faced, her pale blue sweater covered with crumbled leaves, her white jeans smeared with dirt.

After three weeks of this, my mother, who is a musician and widely regarded as eccentric, said to my father, who is a psychiatrist and a kind, sad man, "She's going off."

"What is that, your professional opinion?" He picked up the newspaper and put it down again, sighing. "I'm sorry, I didn't mean to snap at you. I know something's bothering her. Have you talked to her?"

"What's there to say? David, she's going crazy. She doesn't need a heart-to-heart talk with Mom, she needs a hospital."

They went back and forth, and my father sat down with Rose for a few hours, and she sat there licking the hairs on her forearm, first one way, then the other. My mother stood in the hallway, dry-eyed and pale, watching the two of them. She had already packed, and when three of my father's friends dropped by to offer free consultations and recommendations, my mother and Rose's suitcase were already in the car. My mother hugged me and told me that they would be back that night, but not with Rose. She also said, divining my worst fear, "It won't happen to you, honey. Some people go crazy and some people never do. You never will." She smiled and stroked my hair. "Not even when you want to."

Rose was in hospitals, great and small, for the next ten years. She had lots of terrible therapists and a few good ones. One place had no pictures on the walls, no windows, and the patients all wore slippers with the hospital crest on them. My mother didn't even bother to go to Admissions. She turned Rose around and the two of them marched out, my father walking behind them, apologizing to his colleagues. My mother ignored the psychiatrists, the social workers, and the nurses, and played Handel and Bessie Smith for the patients on whatever was available. At some places, she had a Steinway donated by a grateful, or optimistic, family; at others, she banged out "Gimme a Pigfoot and a Bottle of Beer" on an old, scarred box that hadn't been tuned since there'd been English-speaking physicians on the grounds. My father talked in serious, appreciative tones to the administrators and unit chiefs and tried to be friendly with whoever was managing Rose's case. We all hated the family therapists.

The worst family therapist we ever had sat in a pale green room with us, visibly taking stock of my mother's ethereal beauty and her faded blue t-shirt and girl-sized jeans, my father's rumpled suit and stained tie, and my own unreadable seventeen-year-old fashion statement. Rose was beyond fashion that year, in one of her dancing teddybear smocks and extra-extra-large Celtics sweatpants. Mr. Walker read Rose's file in front of us and then watched in alarm as Rose began crooning, beautifully, and slowly massaging her breasts. My mother and I laughed, and even my father started to smile. This was Rose's usual opening salvo for new therapists.

Mr. Walker said, "I wonder why it is that everyone is so entertained by Rose behaving inappropriately."

Rose burped and then we all laughed. This was the seventh family therapist we had seen, and none of them had lasted very long. Mr. Walker, unfortunately, was determined to do right by us.

"What do you think of Rose's behavior, Violet?" They did this sometimes. In their manual it must say, If you think the parents are too weird, try talking to the sister.

"I don't know. Maybe she's trying to get you to stop talking about her in the third person."

"Nicely put," my mother said.

"Indeed," my father said.

"Fuckin' A," Rose said.

"Well, this is something that the whole family agrees upon," Mr. Walker said, trying to act as if he understood or even liked us.

"That was not a successful intervention, Ferret Face." Rose tended to function better when she was angry. He did look like a blond ferret, and we all laughed again. Even my father, who tried to give these people a chance, out of some sense of collegiality, had given it up.

After fourteen minutes, Mr. Walker decided that our time was up and walked out, leaving us grinning at each other. Rose was still nuts, but at least we'd all had a little fun.

The day we met our best family therapist started out almost as badly. We scared off a resident and then scared off her supervisor, who sent us Dr. Thorne. Three hundred pounds of Texas chili, cornbread, and Lone Star beer, finished off with big black cowboy boots and a small string tie around the area of his neck.

"O frabjous day, it's Big Nut." Rose was in heaven and stopped massaging her breasts immediately.

"Hey, Little Nut." You have to understand how big a man would have to be to call my sister "little." He christened us all, right away. "And it's the good Doctor Nut, and Madame Hickory Nut, 'cause they are the hardest damn nuts to crack, and over here in the overalls and not much else is No One's Nut"—a name that summed up both my sanity and my loneliness. We all relaxed.

Dr. Thorne was good for us. Rose moved into a halfway house whose director loved Big Nut so much that she kept Rose even when Rose went through a period of having sex with everyone who passed her door. She was in a fever for a while, trying to still the voices by fucking her brains out.

Big Nut said, "Darlin', I can't. I cannot make love to every beautiful woman I meet, and furthermore, I can't do that and be your therapist too. It's a great shame, but I think you might be able to find a really nice guy, someone who treats you just as sweet and kind as I would if I were lucky enough to be your beau. I don't want you to settle for less." And she stopped propositioning the crack addicts and the alcoholics and the guys at the shelter. We loved Dr. Thorne.

My father went back to seeing rich neurotics and helped out one day a week at Dr. Thorne's Walk-In Clinic. My mother finished a recording of Mozart concerti and played at fund-raisers for Rose's halfway house. I went back to college and found a wonderful linebacker from Texas to sleep with. In the dark, I would make him call me "darlin'." Rose took her meds, lost about fifty pounds, and began singing at the A.M.E. Zion Church, down the street from the halfway house.

At first they didn't know what to do with this big blond lady, dressed funny and hovering wistfully in the doorway during their rehearsals, but she gave them a few bars of "Precious Lord" and the choir director felt God's hand and saw that with the help of His sweet child Rose, the Prospect Street Choir was going all the way to the Gospel Olympics.

Amidst a sea of beige, umber, cinnamon, and espresso faces, there was Rose, bigger, blonder, and pinker than any two white women could be. And Rose and the choir's contralto, Addie Robicheaux, laid out their gold and silver voices and wove them together in strands as fine as silk, as strong as steel. And we wept as Rose and Addie, in their billowing garnet robes, swayed together, clasping hands until the last perfect note floated up to God, and then they smiled down at us.

Rose would still go off from time to time and the voices would tell her to do bad things, but Dr. Thorne or Addie or my mother could usually bring her back. After five good years, Big Nut died. Stuffing his face with a chili dog, sitting in his unair-conditioned office in the middle of July, he had one big, Texas-sized aneurysm and died.

Rose held on tight for seven days; she took her meds, went to choir practice, and rearranged her room about a hundred times. His funeral was like a Lourdes for the mentally ill. If you were psychotic, borderline, bad-off neurotic, or just very hard to get along with, you were there. People shaking so bad from years of heavy meds that they fell out of the pews.

People holding hands, crying, moaning, talking to themselves. The crazy people and the not-so-crazy people were all huddled together, like puppies at the pound.

Rose stopped taking her meds, and the halfway house wouldn't keep her after she pitched another patient down the stairs. My father called the insurance company and found out that Rose's new, improved psychiatric coverage wouldn't begin for forty-five days. I put all of her stuff in a garbage bag, and we walked out of the halfway house, Rose winking at the poor drooling boy on the couch.

"This is going to be difficult—not all bad, but difficult—for the whole family, and I thought we should discuss everybody's expectations. I know I have some concerns." My father had convened a family meeting as soon as Rose finished putting each one of her thirty stuffed bears in its own special place.

"No meds," Rose said, her eyes lowered, her stubby fingers, those fingers that had braided my hair and painted tulips on my cheeks, pulling hard on the hem of her dirty smock.

My father looked in despair at my mother.

"Rosie, do you want to drive the new car?" my mother asked.

Rose's face lit up. "I'd love to drive that car. I'd drive to California, I'd go see the bears at the San Diego Zoo. I would take you, Violet, but you always hated the zoo. Remember how she cried at the Bronx Zoo when she found out that the animals didn't get to go home at closing?" Rose put her damp hand on mine and squeezed it sympathetically. "Poor Vi."

"If you take your medication, after a while you'll be able to drive the car. That's the deal. Meds, car." My mother sounded accommodating but unenthusiastic, careful not to heat up Rose's paranoia.

"You got yourself a deal, darlin'."

I was living about an hour away then, teaching English during the day, writing poetry at night. I went home every few days for dinner. I called every night.

My father said, quietly, "It's very hard. We're doing all right, I think. Rose has been walking in the mornings with your mother, and she watches a lot of TV. She won't go to the day hospital, and she won't go back to the choir. Her friend Mrs. Robicheaux came by a couple of times. What a sweet woman. Rose wouldn't even talk to her. She just sat there, staring at the wall and humming. We're not doing all that well, actually, but I guess we're getting by. I'm sorry, sweetheart, I don't mean to depress you."

My mother said, emphatically, "We're doing fine. We've got our routine and we stick to it and we're fine. You don't need to come home so often, you know. Wait 'til Sunday, just come for the day. Lead your life, Vi. She's leading hers."

I stayed away all week, afraid to pick up my phone, grateful to my mother for her harsh calm and her reticence, the qualities that had enraged me throughout my childhood.

I came on Sunday, in the early afternoon, to help my father garden, something we had always enjoyed together. We weeded and staked tomatoes and killed aphids while my mother and Rose were down at the lake. I didn't even go into the house until four, when I needed a glass of water.

Someone had broken the piano bench into five neatly stacked pieces and placed them where the piano bench usually was.

"We were having such a nice time, I couldn't bear to bring it up," my father said, standing in the doorway, carefully keeping his gardening boots out of the kitchen.

"What did Mommy say?"

"She said, 'Better the bench than the piano.' And your sister lay down on the floor and just wept. Then your mother took her down to the lake. This can't go on, Vi. We have twenty-seven days left, your mother gets no sleep because Rose doesn't sleep, and if I could just pay twenty-seven thousand dollars to keep her in the hospital until the insurance takes over, I'd do it."

"All right. Do it. Pay the money and take her back to Hartley-Rees. It was the prettiest place, and she liked the art therapy there."

"I would if I could. The policy states that she must be symptom-free for at least forty-five days before her coverage begins. Symptom-free means no hospitalization."

"Jesus, Daddy, how could you get that kind of policy? She hasn't been symptom-free for forty-five minutes."

"It's the only one I could get for long-term psychiatric." He put his hand over his mouth, to block whatever he was about to say, and went back out to the garden. I couldn't see if he was crying.

He stayed outside and I stayed inside until Rose and my mother came home from the lake. Rose's soggy sweatpants were rolled up to her knees, and she had a bucketful of shells and seaweed, which my mother persuaded her to leave on the back porch. My mother kissed me lightly and told Rose to go up to her room and change out of her wet pants.

Rose's eyes grew very wide. "Never. I will never . . ." She knelt down and began banging her head on the kitchen floor with rhythmic intensity, throwing all her weight behind each attack. My mother put her arms around Rose's waist and tried to hold her back. Rose shook her off, not even looking around to see what was slowing her down. My mother lay up against the refrigerator.

"Violet, please . . ."

I threw myself onto the kitchen floor, becoming the spot that Rose was smacking her head against. She stopped a fraction of an inch short of my stomach.

"Oh, Vi, Mommy, I'm sorry. I'm sorry, don't hate me." She staggered to her feet and ran wailing to her room.

My mother got up and washed her face brusquely, rubbing it dry with a dishcloth. My father heard the wailing and came running in, slipping his long bare feet out of his rubber boots.

"Galen, Galen, let me see." He held her head and looked closely for bruises on her pale, small face. "What happened?" My mother looked at me. "Violet, what happened? Where's Rose?"

"Rose got upset, and when she went running upstairs she pushed Mommy out of the way." I've only told three lies in my life, and that was my second.

"She must feel terrible, pushing you, of all people. It would have to be you, but I know she didn't want it to be." He made my mother a cup of tea, and all the love he had for her, despite her silent rages and her vague stares, came pouring through the teapot, warming her cup, filling her small, long-fingered hands. She rested her head against his hip, and I looked away.

"Let's make dinner, then I'll call her. Or you call her, David, maybe she'd rather see your face first."

Dinner was filled with all of our starts and stops and Rose's desperate efforts to control herself. She could barely eat and hummed the McDonald's theme song over and over again, pausing only to spill her juice down the front of her smock and begin weeping. My father looked at my mother and handed Rose his napkin. She dabbed at herself listlessly, but the tears stopped.

"I want to go to bed. I want to go to bed and be in my head. I want to go to bed and be in my bed and in my head and just wear red. For red is the color that my baby wore and once more, it's true, yes, it is, it's true. Please don't wear red tonight, oh, oh, please don't wear red tonight, for red is the color—"

"Okay, okay, Rose. It's okay. I'll go upstairs with you and you can get ready for bed. Then Mommy will come up and say good night too. It's okay, Rose." My father reached out his hand and Rose grasped it, and they walked out of the dining room together, his long arm around her middle.

My mother sat at the table for a moment, her face in her hands, and then she began clearing the plates. We cleared without talking, my mother humming Schubert's "Schlummerlied," a lullaby about the woods and the river calling to the child to go to sleep. She sang it to us every night when we were small.

My father came into the kitchen and signaled to my mother. They went upstairs and came back down together a few minutes later.

"She's asleep," they said, and we went to sit on the porch and listen to the crickets. I don't remember the rest of the evening, but I remember it as quietly sad, and I remember the rare sight of my parents holding hands, sitting on the picnic table, watching the sunset.

I woke up at three o'clock in the morning, feeling the cool night air through my sheet. I went down the hall for a blanket and looked into Rose's room, for no reason. She wasn't there. I put on my jeans and a sweater and went downstairs. I could feel her absence. I went outside and saw her wide, draggy footprints darkening the wet grass into the woods.

"Rosie," I called, too softly, not wanting to wake my parents, not wanting to startle Rose. "Rosie, it's me. Are you here? Are you all right?"

I almost fell over her. Huge and white in the moonlight, her flowered smock bleached in the light and shadow, her sweatpants now completely wet. Her head was flung back, her white, white neck exposed like a lost Greek column.

"Rosie, Rosie—" Her breathing was very slow, and her lips were not as pink as they usually were. Her eyelids fluttered.

"Closing time," she whispered. I believe that's what she said.

I sat with her, uncovering the bottle of white pills by her hand, and watched the stars fade.

When the stars were invisible and the sun was warming the air, I went back to the house. My mother was standing on the porch, wrapped in a blanket, watching me. Every step I took overwhelmed me; I could picture my mother slapping me, shooting me for letting her favorite die.

"Warrior queens," she said, wrapping her thin strong arms around me. "I raised warrior queens." She kissed me fiercely and went into the woods by herself.

Later in the morning she woke my father, who could not go into the woods, and still later she called the police and the funeral parlor. She hung up the phone, lay down, and didn't get back out of bed until the day of the funeral. My father fed us both and called the people who needed to be called and picked out Rose's coffin by himself.

My mother played the piano and Addie sang her pure gold notes and I closed my eyes and saw my sister, fourteen years old, lion's mane thrown back and eyes tightly closed against the glare of the parking lot lights. That sweet sound held us tight, flowing around us, eddying through our hearts, rising, still rising.

## The Mother-in-Law
Doris Betts

I cross the alley which runs between the back of the neighborhood grocery and the back of *her* house. I believe it is 1932. Now softly to the
lighted bedroom window to part the dry spirea twigs and see through the
cloudy pane.

Already yellowing, she rests in the high bed and breathes through her
mouth. She is barely forty and her heart does not want to stop; it beats
against the cancer like a fist on a landslide.

They sit around her bed. Husband, three sons. Another long evening.
They talk over the day like any ordinary family.

There is the youngest boy, Philip. Black eyes and silence. In ten more
years, he will marry me.

She does not ask them the only question which still concerns her: Will
you look after Ross? So they do not answer. If I could slip into the room
and make her hear, I would whisper, "Yes, of course"; but she has never
heard of me, and never will.

I am a ghost here and my other self is skipping rope in another state.

Snow on the alley. Nathan, the eldest, hangs back. He feels responsible for
everything he sees, and started living through a long lens at an early age.
Ahead of him, Ross is scraping fingers in the snow, slinging handfuls
behind him. My future husband walks sideways, so he can look ahead and
watch Ross at the same time. He lacks Nathan's sense of duty; with him,
all is instinct.

They come to the rear of the grocery store, where trucks unload at

Doris Betts, "The Mother-in-Law," from *Beasts of the Southern Wild and Other Stories.* ©
1973 by Doris Betts and HarperCollins Publishers, Inc. Reprinted by permission of Russell &
Volkening as agents for Doris Betts.

the ramp and fermenting produce is piled in cans. Since the woolen mill closed, the cans rattle all night. People trot up the alley carrying tow sacks.

With his good arm, Ross makes a snowball spatter on their empty garage. The car has been sold. Nathan tries to decide whether the thump disturbs their mother. My husband throws snow, too, and makes his ball fall short. By instinct.

Nathan stops, points. Above the loading ramp, the grocer has installed two poles with electric lights which will shine directly on the garbage cans. Now the boys must keep their window shades pulled at night to avoid recognizing the fathers of friends.

They turn in the sagging wire gate to their back yard. Under the snow lie *her* crowded iris; the stalks of uncut chrysanthemums rattle when Ross limps through. Nathan reaches out to help him across a drift. Before he can grasp the hand, my future husband has dropped snow down Ross' back; they roll and tussle. Philip gets wetter. A draw—Ross laughs. I am watching the scene with my own hand out; if I were to change this or that?

They walk through my transparent arm and climb the back steps. The pattern is set.

Mr. Felts has asked the grocer not to burn his big lights all night long. "They shine in her window." She sleeps so little now, even with medicine. All night he hears the "sooo—soooo" as she sucks breath through her clenched teeth.

The grocer says the police advised it. His windows, door locks are being broken. Obliquely he blames Mr. Felts for the Depression, because he is an accountant and is still working the town's math when its weaving machines have stopped.

The grocer's son ran a machine. "I better leave them on."

Mr. Felts fastens her window shade with thumbtacks. Still the gold leaks in. The shine frightens her; she knows the back alley has never been bright. If there is a fire, Ross will not be able to get away.

Again Mr. Felts begs the grocer. Those who raid the garbage cans do it hastily now, half blinded, in a clatter. She hears; she sucks air faster. One night a metal lid rolls down the entire alley and spins out with a twang against the corner curb. She—who never missed church until this illness— cries out about Ezekiel's chariot.

Next morning, in full sight of the neighborhood, Mr. Felts heaves bricks at the light until both bulbs are broken. He wants to throw one at the grocer, too, but Nathan stops him.

March. When they come home from the funeral, Ross hurries to the bedroom. He does not understand she will not lie there anymore. Only Nathan was old enough to see inside the box. He takes Ross now onto the back steps and speaks for a long time about death and Heaven. Ross hits him.

In her bedroom, their father pulls outward gently on the shade. One by one, the thumbtacks pop onto the floor like buttons off a fat man. My husband smiles when he sees this; my ghost smiles. How I am going to love him!

Crying at last, Ross slams the back door and screams his name.

"Come here," Philip says. "Help me pick up these tacks."

Ross was born with a bad arm and leg. One eye is fixed and useless; there is slight vision in the other. While there was money, the Felts saw many doctors. Casts and splints were used; his night brace banged the bars of the crib when he dreamed.

His spectacles are plain glass and thick glass, so his brain seems to be bulging out through the magnified eye which strains to see shapes, light, and shadow. Ross is intelligent and, thanks to *her*, well adjusted. She must have bitten her tongue half off the day he climbed onto the garage roof. How her throat swelled shut the first of the hundred times he fell downstairs. But she was successful. All boys fall, Ross thinks.

Summer evenings there was baseball in the vacant lot by the grocer's. Ross batted like a spider, ran bases like a crab. The boys' laughter sounded to him like comradeship. In the bull pen Nathan made sure it was. Philip told me these things.

Now that I have Philip's children, I know how many bloody noses she iced in the pantry. I go into that pantry and watch her from behind the flour bin. She is thinking about the first lumps which have bent her nipple. I understand why she's sure they are harmless; it is not her *turn* for cancer. At night I tap my foot silently by the green chair while she searches her Bible. I'm not a Bible reader myself. I like the Greek myths. She reads St. Paul.

Staring at the green chair, where in more than a decade my other self will sit, she almost meets my eyes, almost pledges to accept any unbeliever who will care for Ross.

"I'm going to be pretty and red-haired," I say—she doesn't care.

"In bed, Philip and I . . ." She can't be bothered.

She dreams beyond me of how Ross kicked against her womb with a foot that could not have been withered. It was Achilles' foot.

Nathan, the dutiful son, has brought her daisies, which she puts absently into a vase. I beg her: Look at my Philip now. He carries no flowers but his black eyes—does she see? Now she embraces Ross and, over his crooked shoulder, gazes deeply at her other sons. She cannot help it; she has begun to bargain. Will they? Can they? Has she prepared them to?

Harmless as marbles, the fragments of her death shift in her breast and another, smaller, rolls in the womb that sheltered Ross and the others. I, Nathan's wife, their children, ours—we hear the bits roll as she looks through time and our faces.

She lets Ross go; the moment passes, will exist in no one's memory but hers and mine.

In 1942, Nathan becomes an army officer. Philip is in high school, unaware that in another state I am in love with a basketball center who owns his own car. We park in it, too; I evade his long arms. Philip's ghost sits in the back seat. I sense him there. I am uneasy, dimly suspecting he exists, fearing his shade is nothing but my frigidity.

This is the year Mr. Felts has almost finished paying the cost of her futile treatment—X-rays and pills—the headstone. He shrinks as the bills shrink; his flesh seems to drain away toward hers. Philip says, "You rest, I'll read tonight." Ross is a college freshman. They take turns with his texts.

The grocery store has been torn down and a warehouse built. Its lights shine day and night, and light up the place in her yard where the iris roots have reared up to lie on the ground like a tumble of potatoes.

At fifteen, I go away to girls' camp in the Blue Ridge Mountains. My parents can afford it. Across the same lake, their church holds summer retreat. Mr. Felts has brought the two younger boys because he promised her. In the dark, Philip smokes secretly after hours and stares over the black water at the lights of the camp where I am sleeping. I can't see what Mr. Felts is doing.

Once, on my horse, I ride across the place where Philip and Ross have had a picnic; they have just gone; maybe no more than a rhododendron bush keeps us from meeting.

Up the hill as they walk away, Ross is asking, "Isn't it time you got interested in girls?"

Now it's time. I go to college in his town. I am eighteen, so ignorant and idealistic that the qualities overlap and blend. My grades are good. I think I will become a social worker and improve the world. I sign up to read for blind students.

(Here I must pause. The ghost of my English teacher protests such melodrama, such coincidence. I, too, protest it. I am a tool of the plot, a flat character rung in on the proper page. I say—with Iphigenia—thanks but no thanks! The blade comes on.)

In no time at all, I move from knowing Ross to knowing Philip. I recognize him. He looks like his mother. While we are falling in love, we take Ross everywhere with us. He can ride a gentle mare, swim an awkward backstroke. In the balcony, we explain movie scenes if the dialogue is vague. He hardly notices when we kiss or touch each other. One night, drunk and tired of trying to work out marriage plans, we let Ross drive down a country road—screaming directions, "Right!" and "Left!"—till all three of us hurt from laughing. I kiss Philip so hard my own teeth bite me.

Secretly, Ross talks to me about wanting girls. I repeat it to Philip, whose black eyes go blacker. Nathan is mailing long letters home about how Ross should save himself for his bride.

In spite of what the basketball center said, I am not frigid. Lost at last under Philip, Philip lost in me. In the silence afterward, the ghost of Ross. We get up and dress and go find him and take him for a long walk. Coming home, we sit with our backs against the warehouse, singing. Soprano, tenor, baritone, under the blazing lights.

We marry and the war ends. Ross has a job running a machine he can pedal with one foot. With his checks he buys radios and phonographs. Every morning, Mr. Felts cooks him Cream of Wheat.

Philip and I live over a beauty shop. The smell of hot hair has got into our linens. Philip finishes college; Nathan comes home and begins.

Saturday nights I go to her house and cook a big pot of spaghetti. I am pregnant with our first. Philip is independent and we have refused to cash my parents' checks, which have grown smaller anyway.

I wash the dishes in her sink. Did she cook spaghetti here? Ross likes it. Yes.

Late in the evening when my back aches, I leave the men talking and lie across her bed. They have painted the window sill, but its frame is neatly pocked where the shade was nailed down. I lie there fearful for my child.

I ask her: What were the earliest signs? Did you vomit much? Take vitamins?

But she has slipped into the room where Ross and the others are playing cards.

Our daughter is almost ready for kindergarten. The next one is walking and throwing toys; the third sleeps through the night at last. I have got used to the beauty-shop smell.

The telephone rings. Ross says, "I came in? The coffee wasn't fixed?"

I call to our bedroom, "Philip?"

In my ear the telephone: "I can't find where he's gone."

"I'll come," Philip says.

They find Mr. Felts in the furnace room. The shovel is under the coal, and he has gone down around its handle like a wilted vine. His heart tried to get out; all is stained.

We bring Ross home to our four rooms. Afterward I visit her empty house. Where are you, Mr. Felts? What was it like for you? Why did you never say?

Silence. He was as still as Philip is.

Ross lives with us now. Nathan fills out his income tax. He buys insurance policies for Ross. He never forgets a birthday and they ask Ross to dinner once a month. Nathan's daughters go to orthodontists and reducing salons.

I carry four baskets of laundry up these stairs instead of three. Our children like bread pudding. All four are healthy, make noise, eat a lot. They will have straighter teeth when the second set comes in.

Philip works too hard. Some Saturday nights he sits in the kitchen and drinks whiskey alone until his own limbs seem crippled. I have to help him down the hall. "Something worrying you?"

"What could be worrying me?"

I have stopped asking. What he cannot say, I must not. Mostly we talk over our days like any ordinary family.

Sometimes when our bedspring has stopped squeaking, I can hear Ross's squeak. Do the children hear? What will we do when they are too old to share his room? He never complains of the sweat when the vaporizer steams all night and I come in and out with aspirin. Sometimes he sits up in bed to smoke and wait. I'm afraid he'll set the mattress afire some night when I sleep through the smoke.

"Let me light you a cigarette," he always offers.

I always let him. Philip says Ross needs to give us something back.

Lung cancer? I never say that aloud. Secretly, I flush the butt down the toilet.

"I've got more," Ross always calls pleasantly when I come back into the hall.

Now, while the children sleep and Ross sleeps among them and I sit down at last to wait for Philip to come from his overtime work, somebody rattles my garbage can; somebody breathes on my glass, looking in. Somebody's glance like a blaze of light gets under my shade.

I am mending *his* shirt. I am forty, like *her.*

I say to the black windowpane: Yes, we are. Go away.

She understands and her gaze burns past to where Ross still sleeps in a brace in the crib she bought. I understand her, too. Even on weary nights, I am glad her desire found me, drew me to this room.

He's just fine, I say. He will live a long life.

Then, for one icy moment, the ghost of her envy stares at the ghost of mine.

# PART II

**The Culture
of Medicine and the
Physician-Patient
Relationship**

## Basic Clinical Skills: The First Encounters
Melvin Konner

For some students in medical school, the ultimate encounter with the patient is not essentially new. This includes the few students who were previously nurses or physician associates and the larger number who have volunteered extensively to work in hospital or other clinical settings. But for many if not most, this experience is the most keenly anticipated and most anxious moment of life as a medical student.

Almost all medical students are young enough so that the naive energy of youth overcomes any natural timidity. To extend the analogy of the adolescent crush, contact with a patient, like marriage, is easier to get into when you are young and, if not foolish, then at least confident, even headstrong. The older you get the more you know, and after a certain point you know too much; you can envision the pitfalls, and you feel embarrassed by what earlier might have been a rough but effective brash éclat. I noticed in myself a level of concern about how I would handle patients, how they would react to me, what I might do wrong that, if not exactly inappropriate, was also not perfectly adaptive. I wanted to be the sort of person who would simply dive in, as so many did all around me.

For example, in a moving clinical exercise during the preclinical years, we visited a rehabilitation hospital for a lecture on the subject of paraplegia by a specialist who was a paraplegic himself—the result of an injury that had taken place within weeks of his graduation from medical school. As might be expected, he remarked on many aspects of day-to-day care, the sort that most physicians prefer to relegate to nurses, with a sensitivity and sympathy that few other physicians could have had. Between the lecture and the patient presentations, we took a break, and as we filed out into the hall to stretch our legs, I saw that one of the patients to be presented—a new quadriplegic—was lying on a portable bed in the hallway. He could not have been more than twenty-one or twenty-two. He was handsome, healthy-looking—his muscles had not had time to deteriorate—and had, as the cliché goes, his whole life ahead of him. Yet he had just lost, permanently, the use of his body below the shoulders. I was one of about forty medical students milling around, spilling out of the classroom into the hallway, all healthy, ambitious and strong; and here, uncomfortably close to me, was a young man about as broken as one could be.

I could not think of anything to say to him. Surely this was a situation in which the wrong words could do damage, and I was highly conscious of the power of my embryonic medical role. I had not been taught the right words, so I was reluctant to say any. Still, the awkwardness of the situation as it was could not be much better than even the wrong words, and I began to grope for some phrases that might be acceptable, that might break the barrier.

During the few seconds that I was preoccupied with this effort, one of my fellow students—a particularly uninspiring athletic type, I thought—walked up to the stretcher, looked down at the crippled young man, and said, "Pretty tough break."

Ouch, I thought. Just the sort of thing I wanted to avoid. "Yeah," said the patient, his face brightening perceptibly.

"How did it happen?" the medical student asked, and they began a conversation in which all the barriers I had envisioned immediately broke down. The emotional topology of the hallway, which for me had been dominated by tension resulting from the lack of communication between the medical students and the patient, had been utterly changed.

I was reminded of the advice I once got as a boy about talking to a girl at a party: if she wants to talk to you, it doesn't much matter what you say first; and if she doesn't want to, it doesn't matter either. Unlike the girls of my youth, however, patients almost always want to be spoken to by doctors (including medical students), but it is not so easy to say the wrong thing. Thus I learned from one of my less inspiring fellow medical students the first lesson of interacting with patients: the doctor is not entitled to be reluctant. However awkward the situation, however discouraging or confusing or ugly the disease, however apparently withdrawn the patient, the doctor must step across the barrier in interpersonal space that everyone else must properly respect.

And yet it was plain to see that the result of this forthrightness was not always good. Teachers and students alike "dove in" with a brusque, abrupt style that many patients disliked. The laying on of hands was reduced to the carrying out of procedures, and words exchanged with the patient were basically viewed as tools to make those procedures go more smoothly.

At my medical school it was arranged for first-year students to have preliminary clinical experiences in hospital settings. I was assigned to a small group led by an immigrant physician who happened to be a superb if slightly pompous neurologist. He used to say, "Touch the patient." This, he explained, was a categorical imperative. No matter what, find an excuse to touch the patient, however reluctant you are, however reluctant you imagine the patient is. If necessary, pretend to check for a fever by putting your hand on the patient's forehead. Take an unnecessary pulse. His words made an indelible impression on me.

On this occasion we stepped out of the elevator onto one of the highest floors of a just-finished hospital tower, a surgical ward so new it seemed to glitter. As we turned a corner into the main part of the ward, we saw and became part of a white-coated commotion around a stretcher. My clinical tutor, as the neurologist was called, introduced me to a young woman who was a third-year medical student engaged in her surgical clerkship. Moans were emanating from within the crowd of hospital whites. The medical student narrated the scene in a cheery lilting tone with a bright, fresh expression on her face; but I was riveted by the moans, which were now taking the shape of the word "Mama," pathetically repeated over and over again. The patient was an old-looking woman (I would now characterize her, in retrospect, as merely middle-aged) who was described as an alcoholic and evidently not *compos mentis*. She was undergoing the procedure of placement of a central line—the insertion of a large-bore needle in a major vein below the clavicle—needed for the pouring in of great volumes of fluid, as well as nutrients and drugs.

The woman did not stop moaning, "Mama, Mama, Mama." (I still cannot get those moans out of my mind. One sees terrible things in medicine, and this was far from the worst I saw, but it was my very first encounter as a student in a hospital; I remember it with the vividness that seems to be preserved for first encounters.) She was frail and small, with a long tangle of orange hair. Curled in the fetal position in a faded yellow hospital gown, she kept repeating her epithet like an uncalm mantra. She was surrounded by large sturdy young men, all handsome and strong of voice. They unfolded her brusquely and efficiently from the fetal curl. Her moans became louder and pierced their moderate, if spirited, professional exchanges: "Mama, Mama, Mama, Mama." Glancing off these was the voice of the cheery young medical student whose explanatory commentary I found harder and harder to listen to. I had a thought that I was to have innumerable times over the next few years, although the feeling that went with it would wane: *Why doesn't somebody touch her forehead? Why doesn't somebody take her hand? Why doesn't somebody say, "It's all right"?*

After a deftly conducted struggle in which the woman's resistance was treated as an annoyance and her cries were ignored, the central line was placed and the residents congratulated one another, as they often and properly do. After all, they are learning, and they deserve and need the praise that goes with new achievement. Also, the central line was for this patient a lifeline, and they could breathe that sigh of relief that comes when, as in a movie, we see a drowning person finally grab hold of a rope.

The patient's body recurled into the fetal position, as the young men stepped away from the stretcher. I was close enough so that without being obtrusive (and they were through with her anyway) I could satisfy my strong urge to touch her. At no point did she stop repeating the plaintive cry, "Mama." "It's OK, dear, it's all right," I said, taking her hand and stroking her hair back away from her forehead. She made no obvious response to these gestures, and I naturally thought they might be useless; but that did not mean I should not be making them. Equally, I didn't know whether the residents' matter-of-fact approach to her entered into her experience in any meaningful sense; in retrospect, with greater knowledge of the neuropsychology of brain damage from alcohol and other causes, I can say with some confidence that they didn't know either.

One could wonder, as I shortly did, whether doctors should not maintain a humane approach to patients not only because of the patients themselves but also because of the students and the residents, always likely to act inhumanely because of the stresses of excessive responsibility, overwork, and sleeplessness; or, for the same reason, because of oneself.

This was before I realized that humane acts not directly affecting "care"—a word meaning neither more nor less than medical and surgical intervention for the purpose of favorably altering the course of an illness—are in short supply in the hospital world; that the patient's mental status is only marginally relevant to the effort at helpful verbal or nonverbal communication; and that far from being embarrassed by brusqueness, resi-

dents are more likely to be embarrassed by (and to consider not quite professional) acts and gestures that are other than completely instrumental.

One's shock does not last long, but at that point I was still shocked.
When the residents were gone and the nurses had removed the patient
with her plaintive cries, I looked to the third-year student for some kind of
explanation. "What did you think of that?" I asked her.

"Wasn't that great? You have to see a lot of those before you get a feel for
them. I'll probably get to place a couple of central lines myself before the
clerkship ends."

"Is it difficult to get used to?"

"Oh, it's great, really. The residents are great to you. As long as you do
your scut and keep the patients' labs and everything straight. I love it."

I left with a vision of the brightness in her face and with the lilt of her
voice in my ears, but I was deeply disturbed by what I had seen. On the bus
on the way home I met a psychiatrist whom I had known before I began
medical school. I told her about my experience, and she was moderately
sympathetic to my concern. But I was looking for something stronger,
some sharing of my "obviously" just and righteous anger. The incident
was not a surprise to her, and although she deplored it, she seemed to
accept it and to consider my reaction somewhat immature, surprisingly
so, given my relatively advanced age.

"That's just the way things are," was about what she had to offer. When
I confided that I might decide I couldn't be a part of this, she did not take
me very seriously. "You'll get used to it," she said. "You don't have to
become like them." She left me with the sensible advice that whatever
was going on around you, you could and should be the way you wanted to
be. "Light your corner," she said finally and emphatically.

We had many good discussions, formal and informal. Our teachers were
strongly oriented to clinical work and were concerned about psychological and ethical aspects of the doctor-patient relationship. (I did not grasp at
the time how unusual this was, and my appreciation of what I was getting
was blunted by the erroneous assumption that it was characteristic of
clinical training in general.)

In this setting I learned a lot about myself. For example, in one exercise
we were given the following problem. A patient needs a kidney transplant. Family members are immunologically surveyed, and a brother is
found who can be a technically successful donor. The brother is con-
fidentially interviewed and refuses. The patient is told that no suitable

donor is available, "suitability" being understood to include technical factors as well as willingness to donate. I argued strongly that the patient should have been told that his brother was immunologically eligible and had refused to donate; otherwise seeds of suspicion with respect to the whole family might have been sown in the patient's mind. The brother, I thought, should be made to take the consequences of his refusal.

Later I had second thoughts and decided that I had spoken glibly. Kidney donation is a risky enterprise, and it is not at all clear that one owes such a bodily sacrifice to anyone, even a brother. Also, kidney transplants often do not work, and the potential uselessness of the sacrifice cannot be ignored. I did not change my mind exactly. I simply made the single most important discovery one can make about such problems, confirmed many times since: they have no right answer. My appreciation of that fact increased with further clinical encounters. The proposition has a corollary: *whatever* a doctor does in such a situation, it can be viewed from the outside as having been the wrong choice. It is only by living through the anguish of such choices that we come to appreciate the ethical depths they sound.

We had a number of introductory lectures on clinical topics, and the most important of these concerned various aspects of history-taking and physical examination, in support of the complete histories and physicals we were doing regularly. As I had been before, I was a bit diffident in these encounters, finding it hard to cross the conventional barriers to interpersonal interaction that I had built up over half a lifetime. It was especially difficult for me to ask patients questions about their use of alcohol and about their sex lives, subjects we were expected to probe deeply, skeptically, and efficiently. This was all the more difficult since we were not participating in patient care but were there by sufferance; patients had been (quite properly) asked to give their permission to be interviewed and examined by second-year medical students, for the benefit of our education.

My first encounter was comically awkward. Purely by chance, I was assigned to a woman who told me during the brief interview that she was an actress with a local repertory company, the name of which I recognized. She was twenty-two years old, had long auburn hair and large brown eyes, and, although small, carried herself with considerable bearing. She had presence—despite being in the hospital, on a bed, dressed in a drab hospital gown. She was about to be discharged, but her physicians had failed to find the source of the pain she still had, a moderate fluctuating sharp discomfort in the lower left quadrant of her abdomen.

She was not in pain at that moment, and at its worst the pain was not very great, but her poise was noticeably disturbed by worry. She had been talked into letting a student do this examination, and it was the last thing she had to do before leaving the hospital. My charge was to give her a complete *neurological* examination. This was utterly irrelevant to her problem; but it was deemed a good way for me to begin, being the most methodical and meticulous part of the physical examination and the easiest to relate meaningfully to anatomy and physiology. One proceeded literally from head to toe, testing sensation, muscle tone and strength, reflexes, perceptual discrimination and integration, and finally higher coordination of movement and thought.

As in most neurological examinations, there was no reason to intrude on any part of the body ordinarily considered intimate, and of course I did not. But I soon found out that any part of the body is intimate in the sense that it is protected by the customary barriers of interpersonal space. There are cultures where these barriers are fewer or lighter than they are for us, and others where they are more numerous or severe. But they are always definite and somehow are known to every person in the culture, if only subconsciously. A violation of these strictures, subtle as they may seem, can dramatically transform the nature of a relationship—resulting in embarrassment, in ostracism, in legal action, or even in homicide. Anthropologists had discovered that diplomatic and business failures—for example, in Japan or in Arab countries—may sometimes be traced to missteps in the frame of personal space.

Yet the physician is supposed to cross these barriers briskly, with confidence and aplomb. And the medical student crossing them for the first time must pretend to the same confidence, ignoring the force and weight of all the previous years of obscure but strict training with regard to personal space. I certainly did try to pretend, and my task was greatly complicated by the fact that I was doing my very first physical examination on a woman who promptly aroused in me unmistakable if fleeting feelings of romantic tenderness and sexual desire. I could not imagine that she was unaware of this, and so another dimension of intersubjectivity was added to an already complex interaction.

I was desperately trying to produce from memory the obsessive protracted sequence of the neurological examination, trying to appear professional, trying to conceal (at all costs!) the fact that I had never examined a patient before (which was probably transparently obvious), and trying to carry forward a stream of small talk, all the while suppressing ridiculous lustful sentiments. The simplest things—looking into her mouth, testing the suppleness of her neck, pushing down on her knee to test the muscle strength in her thighs, checking the mobility of her ankle joint—seemed almost intolerably intrusive. Touching the neck or the knee of a beautiful woman was something one earned with an appropriate investment of time and sentiment: candlelight dinners, walks in the moonlight, that sort of thing (or at least, in this age of marvels, a couple of drinks in a singles bar). But to the patient, I was just one of a long line of men and women who had come around to poke at her in the service of various obscure hospital purposes. She understood perfectly well that the rules of interpersonal space are totally different in a medical encounter; it was I who had trouble with the contrast. Understandably, there were moments when the poor young woman almost burst out laughing.

Later I confided my feelings to the group, with the encouragement of the doctor who was leading that day's discussion. He was a very well-meaning man who was appropriately sensitive—indeed almost too much so. (People who say "share" more than twice in one conversation are always suspect to me, and he exceeded this limit by some measure.) He was trying rather desperately to elicit some valuable confessions about our first experience of the physical examination and not getting very far, so I decided to help him out—having been a teacher, I was alert for those moments when panic is setting in because of student unresponsiveness. I said rather flatly that I had had to examine a woman who was very attractive, and that this made me uncomfortable. There was no response from any of my fellow students, who looked at me strangely. "Thank you for sharing that with us," Dr. Clark finally said, and went on to the next topic. I now knew that this was not to be a forum for discussion about learning to be a doctor, as had been claimed, but yet another setting in which everything about you, even feelings, would be judged. I became accordingly diffident about my feelings.

At this time I seemed to be what I came to call "medically accident-prone." Amusingly, ironically, and probably not entirely coincidentally, I found myself in life situations where my nascent skills seemed to be called for. The first time was on the airplane on the way back from Edinburgh, where I had spoken at a World Health Organization conference on breast-feeding. The pilot's voice scratched over the public address system asking if there were a medical doctor among the passengers. I held my breath for a while, then asked a stewardess what was up. A middle-aged passenger had collapsed, and they feared a heart attack. I was certainly no doctor, but I was feeling the squeeze of responsibility. If I opened my mouth would it do more harm than good? Fortunately, I did not have to answer the question: there were two physicians aboard.

A week or so later I had been attending an intolerably tedious anthropological lecture in a stuffy lecture hall. I had been on the way home from the hospital and still had my little bag with me—it was the only time during medical school when we actually carried those bags—and I was trying to hide it under my seat. The lecturer droned and ostentatiously turned his pages. The air in the room was so thick it was difficult to breathe. As we filed out, I noticed a commotion and saw that a young woman had fainted. Some people got her to a bench, and I rolled up her coat and put it under her legs. She was soon awake, complaining of a pain in her eye, which I tried to examine gently. "I'm a second-year medical student," I said. "I'm not going to touch your eye, but if you like I can look at it." She said that when she fainted she had scratched her eye on her glasses. The eye was teary but looked intact, except for what seemed to be a scratch on the surface of the sclera—the membrane covering the white. She said that she had an ophthalmologist in town, and I offered to call him. I told her to stay where she was.

He was not terribly excited by my story. He said he would see her at his office in an hour. I tried to get him to tell me how worried I should be, and he tried to be noncommittal. "Take a history," he said. There was no revelant history, as was obvious from what I had already told him. So I simply stayed with her until she got a ride home with her parents. I had judged that this was not an emergency, and I was right.

The third incident, a week or two after that, involved a "consultation" by the rather reckless twenty-four-year-old son of an old friend of mine. The young man, who in every way still acted like a teenage boy, was using the injectable anesthetic ketamine, not a "conventional" street drug. He wanted me to provide him with information about it. I looked over the package insert, already stunned. What I found out was not at all reassuring. Ketamine had a low therapeutic ratio, which meant that the difference between an effective dose and a lethal dose was not very great. For the dreamlike state and occasional hallucinations that were its incidental side effects, he was risking respiratory depression and potentially fatal cardiac arrhythmias. I warned him strongly about these effects, but he did not seem to take my warning very seriously.

After some thought, I told his father about the episode. The young man was living at home and consistently behaved immaturely. His father was always getting him out of trouble. And he was a close friend. I thought that it was important for him to know.

I discussed all three episodes with my preceptors in Basic Clinical Skills. In their estimation I had done the right thing only once, with the young woman in the lecture hall. On the plane, they said, I should have offered to help in any way I could, introduced myself as a second-year medical student, and described the limitations on my knowledge—ludicrously limited, really. I might have been the closest thing to a doctor on the plane, and I was therefore on the spot. I had to get used to that sense of responsibility.

As for my friend's son, they thought I had taken a serious legal risk. He was an adult and was consulting me about a private medical matter. It was a completely privileged communication. For telling my friend his father about the consultation, he could have sued me, probably successfully.

These events made me understand for the first time that my role in life was going to be permanently changed—no, that it had already been changed. I had to begin to relate to the world as a doctor, because that was the way the world would now be relating to me. That entailed the ready acceptance of heavy responsibility, with all its practical, legal, and social consequences. I was no longer just a passenger, or a member of the audience, or a friend. Within and above all those social roles, I was more and more like a physician.

My first surgical experience made a strong impression on me. I was seeing patients one morning with a general surgeon who was conducting his usual clinic, evaluating patients before surgery or following their progress after it. At around noon he said he had to leave to go to a small hospital on the other side of town where a patient was waiting to have an axillary lymph node biopsy. Since he was coming back afterward, I asked him if he would mind my tagging along, and on the contrary he was pleased. As we rode together he spoke reverentially of the surgeon he had trained under who had inspired him to become a surgeon himself. What had been only a famous name to me now became real, and I felt as if I were in the presence of an authentic, impressive tradition that comprised emotion as well as knowledge and skill.

And ritual. When we arrived at the little hospital, the surgeon—a plump, middle-aged Irishman with no pretensions to the status of his teacher—guided me gently through the procedures of sterile technique. The hand washing was so methodical and repetitive, so exceedingly thorough, that it was like a ritual confirmation of the germ theory, a self-reteaching of that theory, every day. The gowning and gloving were equally ritualistic but more dramatic, since they involved nurses attending the surgeon—and me, his new assistant—like priestesses who, although subordinated, were responsible for the purity of the ritual and who would pounce mercilessly on a technical blemish. I had to put my hands and arms into the gown without letting my fingers contact any part of the front of it. Then I had to plunge my hands, one at a time, into the tight rubber gloves without missing a finger or touching anything or ending up with the fingers too loose. I did my best, as careful as if walking on eggs, and I did not contaminate anything, but the two nurses' pairs of eyes scrutinized me with an unrelenting critical gaze.

The young man on the table was conscious, and his shaved armpit had been prepared with a local anesthetic. I was content to stand and watch, with my rubber-gloved hands gripping each other awkwardly, staying in the sterile area just in front of my chest. The surgeon showed me the lump in the axilla, made his incision, and began quickly and efficiently to explore the wound with his fingers. Suddenly he turned to me. "Put your fingers in and feel it," he said. His own fingers pried the wound open to ease the way for me. There was no avoiding this even if I had wanted to. The young man turned briefly to look at us, but he was not really concerned. I put two fingers of my right hand in and felt in the area where I had seen the shape made by the lump under the skin surface. Timidly, I began to move them around. Finally I felt it, a lump about one centimeter across, smaller than I had expected. I nodded, holding my breath, eye to eye with the surgeon, and removed my hand.

I watched the surgeon take out the offending node and prepare it for pathological study. But that was anticlimactic. I was more interested in the blood on my fingers, the lingering mystery, the feeling in my hand. It was like the feeling or even the smell of a hand used in making love to a woman; my fingers had been inside another person's body, not just in the mouth or the vagina or the rectum, but beneath the protective surface of the skin, the inviolable film set up by millions of years of evolution, the envelope of ultimate individuality. Taking me along with him had been a matter-of-fact random event for the surgeon, but for me it had been an unforgettable experience.

In pediatrics, my supervisor was Ed Gold, who stood out similarly in basic human competence. Pediatricians in general are known for being better people—it sounds silly, but it's true—than most medical specialists. They have accepted the lowest financial status in medicine in exchange for an opportunity to serve in the most nurturant primary care capacity. Ed's touch with children was unsentimental and smooth, but as good as his surname in its ability to calm and even amuse them while he carried out efficiently the necessary examinations and procedures. His handling of parents—the pediatrician's bread and butter—was equally adept. He had worked for a time at the Centers for Disease Control, and he was strongly oriented to preventive medicine.

As a teacher, he managed to confer confidence. He brought out the best in whatever natural skill with children I had, as well as in my experience doing research with children in Africa and my more recent experience as a father. I felt more comfortable with the patients in his consulting room than I had up to then anywhere else in the hospitals and clinics. Toward the end, there was one afternoon when I was closeted for an hour or two with a pair of unusually active ten-year-old twins who were, to use the common expression, bouncing off the walls. I did all that was necessary in interviewing their mother and in observing and examining each of them in turn. I felt in control of the situation and consequently happy.

Ed told me a story that made me appreciate the rigors of internship in a somewhat new and more ominous way. After a long struggle with a deadly illness, he had lost a small child. The parents were grateful to him for the effort—they frequently are—and invited him to their home. They wanted him to be a part of the process of experiencing, and recovering from, their grief. He was touched and was grateful to be with them. They left him alone with a drink in his hand on their living room couch, for a few minutes, while they attended to the dinner they were preparing. He fell asleep, and they left him to sleep, realizing how desperately he needed it.

What struck me was that this unusually sensitive doctor did not have the physical wherewithal to stay awake at such a moment, to serve the function of psychological healing for which he was then badly needed. This was not a man who, in such a situation, would allow himself to fall asleep lightly, and he had felt guilty about it ever since. How bad could the stress of internship be? Worse, evidently, than I had thought.

The parade of exquisitely healthy, normally growing children that came through Ed's clinic, with their usually minor problems, presented a stark contrast to my memory of Africa. That memory in turn made me fear, as it always did, for the health of my own daughter, and of my son who was then soon to be born. Life in general seemed fragile, but children seemed more fragile than anything, and I knew that their basic expectable health and safety was a historical novelty. Not only in Africa but in Europe and the United States a mere century or two before, half of all children could be expected to die.

**Note**

The original has been abridged for this edition.

## The Learning Curve
Atul Gawande

The patient needed a central line. "Here's your chance," S., the chief resident, said. I had never done one before. "Get set up and then page me when you're ready to start."

It was my fourth week in surgical training. The pockets of my short white coat bulged with patient printouts, laminated cards with instructions for doing CPR and reading EKGs and using the dictation system, two surgical handbooks, a stethoscope, wound-dressing supplies, meal tickets, a penlight, scissors, and about a dollar in loose change. As I headed up the stairs to the patient's floor, I rattled.

This will be good, I tried to tell myself: my first real procedure. The patient—fiftyish, stout, taciturn—was recovering from abdominal surgery he'd had about a week earlier. His bowel function hadn't yet returned, and he was unable to eat. I explained to him that he needed intravenous nutrition and that this required a "special line" that would go into his chest. I said that I would put the line in him while he was in his bed, and that it would involve my numbing a spot on his chest with a local anesthetic, and then threading the line in. I did not say that the line was eight inches long and would go into his vena cava, the main blood vessel to his heart. Nor did I say how tricky the procedure could be. There were "slight risks" involved, I said, such as bleeding and lung collapse; in experienced hands, complications of this sort occur in fewer than one case in a hundred.

But, of course, mine were not experienced hands. And the disasters I knew about weighed on my mind: the woman who had died within minutes from massive bleeding when a resident lacerated her vena cava; the man whose chest had to be opened because a resident lost hold of a wire inside the line, which then floated down to the patient's heart; the man who had a cardiac arrest when the procedure put him into ventricular fibrillation. I said nothing of such things, naturally, when I asked the patient's permission to do his line. He said, "OK."

I had seen S. do two central lines; one was the day before, and I'd attended to every step. I watched how she set out her instruments and laid her patient down and put a rolled towel between his shoulder blades to make his chest arch out. I watched how she swabbed his chest with antiseptic, injected lidocaine, which is a local anesthetic, and then, in full sterile garb, punctured his chest near his clavicle with a fat three-inch needle on a syringe. The patient hadn't even flinched. She told me how to avoid hitting the lung ("Go in at a steep angle," she'd said. "Stay *right* under the clavicle"), and how to find the subclavian vein, a branch to the vena cava lying atop the lung near its apex ("Go in at a steep angle. Stay *right* under the clavicle"). She pushed the needle in almost all the way. She drew back on the syringe. And she was in. You knew because the syringe filled with maroon blood. ("If it's bright red, you've hit an artery," she said. "That's not good.") Once you have the tip of this needle poking in the vein, you somehow have to widen the hole in the vein wall, fit the catheter in, and snake it in the right direction—down to the heart, rather than up to the brain—all without tearing through vessels, lung, or anything else.

To do this, S. explained, you start by getting a guide wire in place. She pulled the syringe off, leaving the needle in. Blood flowed out. She picked up a two-foot-long twenty-gauge wire that looked like the steel D string of an electric guitar, and passed nearly its full length through the needle's bore, into the vein, and onward toward the vena cava. "Never force it in," she warned, "and never, ever let go of it." A string of rapid heartbeats fired off on the cardiac monitor, and she quickly pulled the wire back an inch. It had poked into the heart, causing momentary fibrillation. "Guess we're in the right place," she said to me quietly. Then to the patient: "You're doing great. Only a few minutes now." She pulled the needle out over the wire and replaced it with a bullet of thick, stiff plastic, which she pushed in tight to widen the vein opening. She then removed this dilator and threaded the central line—a spaghetti-thick, flexible yellow plastic tube— over the wire until it was all the way in. Now she could remove the wire. She flushed the line with a heparin solution and sutured it to the patient's chest. And that was it.

Today, it was my turn to try. First, I had to gather supplies—a central-line kit, gloves, gown, cap, mask, lidocaine—which took me forever. When I finally had the stuff together, I stopped for a minute outside the patient's door, trying to recall the steps. They remained frustratingly hazy. But I couldn't put it off any longer. I had a page-long list of other things to get done: Mrs. A needed to be discharged; Mr. B needed an abdominal ultrasound arranged; Mrs. C needed her skin staples removed. And every fifteen minutes or so I was getting paged with more tasks: Mr. X was nauseated and needed to be seen; Miss Y's family was here and needed "someone" to talk to them; Mr. Z needed a laxative. I took a deep breath, put on my best don't-worry-I-know-what-I'm-doing look, and went in.

I placed the supplies on a bedside table, untied the patient's gown, and laid him down flat on the mattress, with his chest bare and his arms at his sides. I flipped on a fluorescent overhead light and raised his bed to my height. I paged S. I put on my gown and gloves and, on a sterile tray, laid out the central line, the guide wire, and other materials from the kit. I drew up five cc's of lidocaine in a syringe, soaked two sponge sticks in the yellow-brown Betadine, and opened up the suture packaging.

S. arrived. "What's his platelet count?"

My stomach knotted. I hadn't checked. That was bad: too low and he could have a serious bleed from the procedure. She went to check a computer. The count was acceptable.

Chastened, I started swabbing his chest with the sponge sticks. "Got the shoulder roll underneath him?" S. asked. Well, no, I had forgotten that, too. The patient gave me a look. S., saying nothing, got a towel, rolled it up, and slipped it under his back for me. I finished applying the antiseptic and then draped him so that only his right upper chest was exposed. He squirmed a bit beneath the drapes. S. now inspected my tray. I girded myself.

"Where's the extra syringe for flushing the line when it's in?" Damn. She went out and got it.

I felt for my landmarks. *Here*? I asked with my eyes, not wanting to undermine the patient's confidence any further. She nodded. I numbed the spot with lidocaine. ("You'll feel a stick and a burn now, sir.") Next, I took the three-inch needle in hand and poked it through the skin. I advanced it slowly and uncertainly, a few millimetres at a time. This is a big goddam needle, I kept thinking. I couldn't believe I was sticking it into someone's chest. I concentrated on maintaining a steep angle of entry, but kept spearing his clavicle instead of slipping beneath it.

"Ow!" he shouted.

"Sorry," I said. S. signalled with a kind of surfing hand gesture to go underneath the clavicle. This time, it went in. I drew back on the syringe. Nothing. She pointed deeper. I went in deeper. Nothing. I withdrew the needle, flushed out some bits of tissue clogging it, and tried again.

"Ow!"

Too steep again. I found my way underneath the clavicle once more. I drew the syringe back. Still nothing. He's too obese, I thought. S. slipped on gloves and a gown. "How about I have a look?" she said. I handed her the needle and stepped aside. She plunged the needle in, drew back on the syringe, and, just like that, she was in. "We'll be done shortly," she told the patient.

She let me continue with the next steps, which I bumbled through. I didn't realize how long and floppy the guide wire was until I pulled the coil out of its plastic sleeve, and, putting one end of it into the patient, I very nearly contaminated the other. I forgot about the dilating step until she reminded me. Then, when I put in the dilator, I didn't push quite hard enough, and it was really S. who pushed it all the way in. Finally, we got the line in, flushed it, and sutured it in place.

Outside the room, S. said that I could be less tentative the next time, but that I shouldn't worry too much about how things had gone. "You'll get it," she said. "It just takes practice." I wasn't so sure. The procedure remained wholly mysterious to me. And I could not get over the idea of jabbing a needle into someone's chest so deeply and so blindly. I awaited the X-ray afterward with trepidation. But it came back fine: I had not injured the lung and the line was in the right place.

Not everyone appreciates the attractions of surgery. When you are a medical student in the operating room for the first time, and you see the surgeon press the scalpel to someone's body and open it like a piece of fruit, you either shudder in horror or gape in awe. I gaped. It was not just the blood and guts that enthralled me. It was also the idea that a person, a mere mortal, would have the confidence to wield that scalpel in the first place.

There is a saying about surgeons: "Sometimes wrong; never in doubt." This is meant as a reproof, but to me it seemed their strength. Every day, surgeons are faced with uncertainties. Information is inadequate; the science is ambiguous; one's knowledge and abilities are never perfect. Even with the simplest operation, it cannot be taken for granted that a patient will come through better off—or even alive. Standing at the operating table, I wondered how the surgeon knew that all the steps would go as planned, that bleeding would be controlled and infection would not set in and organs would not be injured. He didn't, of course. But he cut anyway.

Later, while still a student, I was allowed to make an incision myself. The surgeon drew a six-inch dotted line with a marking pen across an anesthetized patient's abdomen and then, to my surprise, had the nurse hand me the knife. It was still warm from the autoclave. The surgeon had me stretch the skin taut with the thumb and forefinger of my free hand. He told me to make one smooth slice down to the fat. I put the belly of the blade to the skin and cut. The experience was odd and addictive, mixing exhilaration from the calculated violence of the act, anxiety about getting it right, and a righteous faith that it was somehow for the person's good. There was also the slightly nauseating feeling of finding that it took more force than I'd realized. (Skin is thick and springy, and on my first pass I did not go nearly deep enough; I had to cut twice to get through.) The moment made me want to be a surgeon—not an amateur handed the knife for a brief moment but someone with the confidence and ability to proceed as if it were routine.

A resident begins, however, with none of this air of mastery—only an overpowering instinct against doing anything like pressing a knife against flesh or jabbing a needle into someone's chest. On my first day as a surgical resident, I was assigned to the emergency room. Among my first patients was a skinny, dark-haired woman in her late twenties who hobbled in, teeth gritted, with a two-foot-long wooden chair leg somehow nailed to the bottom of her foot. She explained that a kitchen chair had collapsed under her and, as she leaped up to keep from falling, her bare foot had stomped down on a three-inch screw sticking out of one of the chair legs. I tried very hard to look like someone who had not got his medical diploma just the week before. Instead, I was determined to be nonchalant, the kind of guy who had seen this sort of thing a hundred times before. I inspected her foot, and could see that the screw was embedded in the bone at the base of her big toe. There was no bleeding and, as far as I could feel, no fracture.

"Wow, that must hurt," I blurted out, idiotically.

The obvious thing to do was give her a tetanus shot and pull out the screw. I ordered the tetanus shot, but I began to have doubts about pulling out the screw. Suppose she bled? Or suppose I fractured her foot? Or something worse? I excused myself and tracked down Dr. W., the senior surgeon on duty. I found him tending to a car-crash victim. The patient was a mess, and the floor was covered with blood. People were shouting. It was not a good time to ask questions.

I ordered an X-ray. I figured it would buy time and let me check my amateur impression that she didn't have a fracture. Sure enough, getting the X-ray took about an hour, and it showed no fracture—just a common screw embedded, the radiologist said, "in the head of the first metatarsal." I showed the patient the X-ray. "You see, the screw's embedded in the head of the first metatarsal," I said. And the plan? she wanted to know. Ah, yes, the plan.

I went to find Dr. W. He was still busy with the crash victim, but I was able to interrupt to show him the X-ray. He chuckled at the sight of it and asked me what I wanted to do. "Pull the screw out?" I ventured. "Yes," he said, by which he meant "Duh." He made sure I'd given the patient a tetanus shot and then shooed me away.

Back in the examining room, I told her that I would pull the screw out, prepared for her to say something like "You?" Instead she said, "OK, Doctor." At first, I had her sitting on the exam table, dangling her leg off the side. But that didn't look as if it would work. Eventually, I had her lie with her foot jutting off the table end, the board poking out into the air. With every move, her pain increased. I injected a local anesthetic where the screw had gone in and that helped a little. Now I grabbed her foot in one hand, the board in the other, and for a moment I froze. Could I really do this? Who was I to presume?

Finally, I gave her a one-two-three and pulled, gingerly at first and then hard. She groaned. The screw wasn't budging. I twisted, and abruptly it came free. There was no bleeding. I washed the wound out, and she found she could walk. I warned her of the risks of infection and the signs to look for. Her gratitude was immense and flattering, like the lion's for the mouse—and that night I went home elated.

In surgery, as in anything else, skill, judgment, and confidence are learned through experience, haltingly and humiliatingly. Like the tennis player and the oboist and the guy who fixes hard drives, we need practice to get good at what we do. There is one difference in medicine, though: we practice on people.

My second try at placing a central line went no better than the first. The patient was in intensive care, mortally ill, on a ventilator, and needed the line so that powerful cardiac drugs could be delivered directly to her heart. She was also heavily sedated, and for this I was grateful. She'd be oblivious of my fumbling.

My preparation was better this time. I got the towel roll in place and the syringes of heparin on the tray. I checked her lab results, which were fine. I also made a point of draping more widely, so that if I flopped the guide wire around by mistake again, it wouldn't hit anything unsterile.

For all that, the procedure was a bust. I stabbed the needle in too shallow and then too deep. Frustration overcame tentativeness and I tried one angle after another. Nothing worked. Then, for one brief moment, I got a flash of blood in the syringe, indicating that I was in the vein. I anchored the needle with one hand and went to pull the syringe off with the other. But the syringe was jammed on too tightly, so that when I pulled it free I dislodged the needle from the vein. The patient began bleeding into her chest wall. I held pressure the best I could for a solid five minutes, but her chest turned black and blue around the site. The hematoma made it impossible to put a line through there anymore. I wanted to give up. But she needed a line and the resident supervising me—a second-year this time— was determined that I succeed. After an X-ray showed that I had not injured her lung, he had me try on the other side, with a whole new kit. I missed again, and he took over. It took him several minutes and two or three sticks to find the vein himself and that made me feel better. Maybe she was an unusually tough case.

When I failed with a third patient a few days later, though, the doubts really set in. Again, it was stick, stick, stick, and nothing. I stepped aside. The resident watching me got it on the next try.

Surgeons, as a group, adhere to a curious egalitarianism. They believe in practice, not talent. People often assume that you have to have great hands to become a surgeon, but it's not true. When I interviewed to get into surgery programs, no one made me sew or take a dexterity test or checked to see if my hands were steady. You do not even need all ten fingers to be accepted. To be sure, talent helps. Professors say that every two or three years they'll see someone truly gifted come through a program—someone who picks up complex manual skills unusually quickly, sees tissue planes before others do, anticipates trouble before it happens. Nonetheless, attending surgeons say that what's most important to them is finding people who are conscientious, industrious, and boneheaded enough to keep at practicing this one difficult thing day and night for years on end. As a former residency director put it to me, given a choice between a ph.d. who had cloned a gene and a sculptor, he'd pick the ph.d. every time. Sure, he said, he'd bet on the sculptor's being more physically talented; but he'd bet on the ph.d.'s being less "flaky." And in the end that matters more. Skill, surgeons believe, can be taught; tenacity cannot. It's an odd approach to recruitment, but it continues all the way up the ranks, even in top surgery departments. They start with minions with no experience in surgery, spend years training them, and then take more of their faculty from these same homegrown ranks.

And it works. There have now been many studies of élite performers—concert violinists, chess grand masters, professional ice-skaters, mathematicians, and so forth—and the biggest difference researchers find between them and lesser performers is the amount of deliberate practice they've accumulated. Indeed, the most important talent may be the talent for practice itself. K. Anders Ericsson, a cognitive psychologist and an expert on performance, notes that the most important role that innate factors play may be in a person's *willingness* to engage in sustained training. He has found, for example, that top performers dislike practicing just as much as others do. (That's why, for example, athletes and musicians usually quit practicing when they retire.) But, more than others, they have the will to keep at it anyway.

I wasn't sure I did. What good was it, I wondered, to keep doing central lines when I wasn't coming close to hitting them? If I had a clear idea of what I was doing wrong, then maybe I'd have something to focus on. But I didn't. Everyone, of course, had suggestions. Go in with the bevel of the needle up. No, go in with the bevel down. Put a bend in the middle of the needle. No, curve the needle. For a while, I tried to avoid doing another line. Soon enough, however, a new case arose.

The circumstances were miserable. It was late in the day, and I'd had to work through the previous night. The patient weighed more than 300 pounds. He couldn't tolerate lying flat because the weight of his chest and abdomen made it hard for him to breathe. Yet he had a badly infected wound, needed intravenous antibiotics, and no one could find veins in his arms for a peripheral iv. I had little hope of succeeding. But a resident does what he is told, and I was told to try the line.

I went to his room. He looked scared and said he didn't think he'd last more than a minute on his back. But he said he understood the situation and was willing to make his best effort. He and I decided that he'd be left sitting propped up in bed until the last possible minute. We'd see how far we got after that.

I went through my preparations: checking his blood counts from the lab, putting out the kit, placing the towel roll, and so on. I swabbed and draped his chest while he was still sitting up. S., the chief resident, was watching me this time, and when everything was ready I had her tip him back, an oxygen mask on his face. His flesh rolled up his chest like a wave. I couldn't find his clavicle with my fingertips to line up the right point of entry. And already he was looking short of breath, his face red. I gave S. a "Do you want to take over?" look. Keep going, she signalled. I made a rough guess about where the right spot was, numbed it with lidocaine, and pushed the big needle in. For a second, I thought it wouldn't be long enough to reach through, but then I felt the tip slip underneath his clavicle. I pushed a little deeper and drew back on the syringe. Unbelievably, it filled with blood. I was in. I concentrated on anchoring the needle firmly in place, not moving it a millimetre as I pulled the syringe off and threaded the guide wire in. The wire fed in smoothly. The patient was struggling hard for air now. We sat him up and let him catch his breath. And then, laying him down one more time, I got the entry dilated and slid the central line in. "Nice job" was all S. said, and then she left.

I still have no idea what I did differently that day. But from then on my lines went in. That's the funny thing about practice. For days and days, you make out only the fragments of what to do. And then one day you've got the thing whole. Conscious learning becomes unconscious knowledge, and you cannot say precisely how.

I have now put in more than a hundred central lines. I am by no means infallible. Certainly, I have had my fair share of complications. I punctured a patient's lung, for example—the right lung of a chief of surgery from another hospital, no less—and, given the odds, I'm sure such things will happen again. I still have the occasional case that should go easily but doesn't, no matter what I do. (We have a term for this. "How'd it go?" a colleague asks. "It was a total flog," I reply. I don't have to say anything more.)

But other times everything unfolds effortlessly. You take the needle. You stick the chest. You feel the needle travel—a distinct glide through the fat, a slight catch in the dense muscle, then the subtle pop through the vein wall—and you're in. At such moments, it is more than easy; it is beautiful.

Surgical training is the recapitulation of this process—floundering followed by fragments followed by knowledge and, occasionally, a moment of elegance—over and over again, for ever harder tasks with ever greater risks. At first, you work on the basics: how to glove and gown, how to drape patients, how to hold the knife, how to tie a square knot in a length of silk suture (not to mention how to dictate, work the computers, order drugs). But then the tasks become more daunting: how to cut through skin, handle the electrocautery, open the breast, tie off a bleeder, excise a tumor, close up a wound. At the end of six months, I had done lines, lumpectomies, appendectomies, skin grafts, hernia repairs, and mastectomies. At the end of a year, I was doing limb amputations, hemorrhoidectomies, and laparoscopic gallbladder operations. At the end of two years, I was beginning to do tracheotomies, small-bowel operations, and leg-artery bypasses.

I am in my seventh year of training, of which three years have been spent doing research. Only now has a simple slice through skin begun to seem like the mere start of a case. These days, I'm trying to learn how to fix an abdominal aortic aneurysm, remove a pancreatic cancer, open blocked carotid arteries. I am, I have found, neither gifted nor maladroit. With practice and more practice, I get the hang of it.

Doctors find it hard to talk about this with patients. The moral burden of practicing on people is always with us, but for the most part it is unspoken. Before each operation, I go over to the holding area in my scrubs and introduce myself to the patient. I do it the same way every time. "Hello, I'm Dr. Gawande. I'm one of the surgical residents, and I'll be assisting your surgeon." That is pretty much all I say on the subject. I extend my hand and smile. I ask the patient if everything is going OK so far. We chat. I answer questions. Very occasionally, patients are taken aback. "No resident is doing my surgery," they say. I try to be reassuring. "Not to worry—I just assist," I say. "The attending surgeon is always in charge."

None of this is exactly a lie. The attending *is* in charge, and a resident knows better than to forget that. Consider the operation I did recently to remove a seventy-five-year-old woman's colon cancer. The attending stood across from me from the start. And it was he, not I, who decided where to cut, how to position the opened abdomen, how to isolate the cancer, and how much colon to take.

Yet I'm the one who held the knife. I'm the one who stood on the operator's side of the table, and it was raised to my six-foot-plus height. I was there to help, yes, but I was there to practice, too. This was clear when it came time to reconnect the colon. There are two ways of putting the ends together—handsewing and stapling. Stapling is swifter and easier, but the attending suggested I handsew the ends—not because it was better for the patient but because I had had much less experience doing it. When it's performed correctly, the results are similar, but he needed to watch me like a hawk. My stitching was slow and imprecise. At one point, he caught me putting the stitches too far apart and made me go back and put extras in between so the connection would not leak. At another point, he found I wasn't taking deep enough bites of tissue with the needle to insure a strong closure. "Turn your wrist more," he told me. "Like this?" I asked. "Uh, sort of," he said.

In medicine, there has long been a conflict between the imperative to give patients the best possible care and the need to provide novices with experience. Residencies attempt to mitigate potential harm through supervision and graduated responsibility. And there is reason to think that patients actually benefit from teaching. Studies commonly find that teaching hospitals have better outcomes than nonteaching hospitals. Residents may be amateurs, but having them around checking on patients, asking questions, and keeping faculty on their toes seems to help. But there is still no avoiding those first few unsteady times a young physician tries to put in a central line, remove a breast cancer, or sew together two segments of colon. No matter how many protections are in place, on average these cases go less well with the novice than with someone experienced.

Doctors have no illusions about this. When an attending physician brings a sick family member in for surgery, people at the hospital think twice about letting trainees participate. Even when the attending insists that they participate as usual, the residents scrubbing in know that it will be far from a teaching case. And if a central line must be put in, a first-timer is certainly not going to do it. Conversely, the ward services and clinics where residents have the most responsibility are populated by the poor, the uninsured, the drunk, and the demented. Residents have few opportunities nowadays to operate independently, without the attending docs scrubbed in, but when we do—as we must before graduating and going out to operate on our own—it is generally with these, the humblest of patients.

And this is the uncomfortable truth about teaching. By traditional ethics and public insistence (not to mention court rulings), a patient's right to the best care possible must trump the objective of training novices. We want perfection without practice. Yet everyone is harmed if no one is trained for the future. So learning is hidden, behind drapes and anesthesia and the elisions of language. And the dilemma doesn't apply just to residents, physicians in training. The process of learning goes on longer than most people know.

I grew up in the small Appalachian town of Athens, Ohio, where my parents are both doctors. My mother is a pediatrician and my father is a urologist. Long ago, my mother chose to practice part time, which she could afford to do because my father's practice became so busy and successful. He has now been at it for more than twenty-five years, and his office is cluttered with the evidence of this. There is an overflowing wall of medical files, gifts from patients displayed everywhere (books, ceramics with Biblical sayings, hand-painted paperweights, blown glass, carved boxes, a figurine of a boy who, when you pull down his pants, pees on you), and, in an acrylic case behind his oak desk, a few dozen of the thousands of kidney stones he has removed.

Only now, as I get glimpses of the end of my training, have I begun to think hard about my father's success. For most of my residency, I thought of surgery as a more or less fixed body of knowledge and skill which is acquired in training and perfected in practice. There was, I thought, a smooth, upward-sloping arc of proficiency at some rarefied set of tasks (for me, taking out gallbladders, colon cancers, bullets, and appendixes; for him, taking out kidney stones, testicular cancers, and swollen prostates). The arc would peak at, say, ten or fifteen years, plateau for a long time, and perhaps tail off a little in the final five years before retirement. The reality, however, turns out to be far messier. You do get good at certain things, my father tells me, but no sooner do you master something than you find that what you know is outmoded. New technologies and operations emerge to supplant the old, and the learning curve starts all over again. "Three-quarters of what I do today I never learned in residency," he says. On his own, fifty miles from his nearest colleague—let alone a doctor who could tell him anything like "You need to turn your wrist more"—he has had to learn to put in penile prostheses, to perform microsurgery, to reverse vasectomies, to do nerve-sparing prostatectomies, to implant artificial urinary sphincters. He's had to learn to use shock-wave lithotripters, electrohydraulic lithotripters, and laser lithotripters (all instruments for breaking up kidney stones); to deploy Double J ureteral stents and Silicone Figure Four Coil stents and Retro-Inject Multi-Length stents (don't even ask); and to maneuver fibre-optic ureteroscopes. All these technologies and techniques were introduced after he finished training. Some of the procedures built on skills he already had. Many did not.

This is the experience that all surgeons have. The pace of medical innovation has been unceasing, and surgeons have no choice but to give the new thing a try. To fail to adopt new techniques would mean denying patients meaningful medical advances. Yet the perils of the learning curve are inescapable—no less in practice than in residency.

For the established surgeon, inevitably, the opportunities for learning are far less structured than for a resident. When an important new device or procedure comes along, as happens every year, surgeons start by taking a course about it—typically a day or two of lectures by some surgical grandees with a few film clips and step-by-step handouts. You take home a video to watch. Perhaps you pay a visit to observe a colleague perform the operation—my father often goes up to the Cleveland Clinic for this. But there's not much by way of hands-on training. Unlike a resident, a visitor cannot scrub in on cases, and opportunities to practice on animals or cadavers are few and far between. (Britain, being Britain, actually bans surgeons from practicing on animals.) When the pulse-dye laser came out, the manufacturer set up a lab in Columbus where urologists from the area could gain experience. But when my father went there the main experience provided was destroying kidney stones in test tubes filled with a urinelike liquid and trying to penetrate the shell of an egg without hitting the membrane underneath. My surgery department recently bought a robotic surgery device—a staggeringly sophisticated $980,000 robot with three arms, two wrists, and a camera, all millimetres in diameter, which, controlled from a console, allows a surgeon to do almost any operation with no hand tremor and with only tiny incisions. A team of two surgeons and two nurses flew out to the manufacturer's headquarters, in Mountain View, California, for a full day of training on the machine. And they did get to practice on a pig and on a human cadaver. (The company apparently buys the cadavers from the city of San Francisco.) But even this was hardly thorough training. They learned enough to grasp the principles of using the robot, to start getting a feel for using it, and to understand how to plan an operation. That was about it. Sooner or later, you just have to go home and give the thing a try on someone.

Patients do eventually benefit—often enormously—but the first few patients may not, and may even be harmed. Consider the experience reported by the pediatric cardiac-surgery unit of the renowned Great Ormond Street Hospital, in London, as detailed in the *British Medical Journal* last April. The doctors described their results from 325 consecutive operations between 1978 and 1998 on babies with a severe heart defect known as transposition of the great arteries. Such children are born with their heart's outflow vessels transposed: the aorta emerges from the right side of the heart instead of the left and the artery to the lungs emerges from the left instead of the right. As a result, blood coming in is pumped right back out to the body instead of first to the lungs, where it can be oxygenated. The babies died blue, fatigued, never knowing what it was to get enough breath. For years, it wasn't technically feasible to switch the vessels to their proper positions. Instead, surgeons did something known as the Senning procedure: they created a passage inside the heart to let blood from the lungs cross backward to the right heart. The Senning procedure allowed children to live into adulthood. The weaker right heart, however, cannot sustain the body's entire blood flow as long as the left. Eventually, these patients' hearts failed, and although most survived to adulthood, few lived to old age.

By the 1980s, a series of technological advances made it possible to do a switch operation safely, and this became the favored procedure. In 1986, the Great Ormond Street surgeons made the changeover themselves, and their report shows that it was unquestionably an improvement. The annual death rate after a successful switch procedure was less than a quarter that of the Senning, resulting in a life expectancy of 63 years instead of 47. But the price of learning to do it was appalling. In their first 70 switch operations, the doctors had a 25% surgical death rate, compared with just 6% with the Senning procedure. Eighteen babies died, more than twice the number during the entire Senning era. Only with time did they master it: in their next 100 switch operations, five babies died.

As patients, we want both expertise and progress; we don't want to acknowledge that these are contradictory desires. In the words of one British public report, "There should be no learning curve as far as patient safety is concerned." But this is entirely wishful thinking.

Recently, a group of Harvard Business School researchers who have made a specialty of studying learning curves in industry decided to examine learning curves among surgeons instead of in semiconductor manufacture or airplane construction, or any of the usual fields their colleagues examine. They followed eighteen cardiac surgeons and their teams as they took on the new technique of minimally invasive cardiac surgery. This study, I was surprised to discover, is the first of its kind. Learning is ubiquitous in medicine, and yet no one had ever compared how well different teams actually do it.

The new heart operation—in which new technologies allow a surgeon to operate through a small incision between ribs instead of splitting the chest open down the middle—proved substantially more difficult than the conventional one. Because the incision is too small to admit the usual tubes and clamps for rerouting blood to the heart-bypass machine, surgeons had to learn a trickier method, which involved balloons and catheters placed through groin vessels. And the nurses, anesthesiologists, and perfusionists all had new roles to master. As you'd expect, everyone experienced a substantial learning curve. Whereas a fully proficient team takes three to six hours for such an operation, these teams took on average three times as long for their early cases. The researchers could not track complication rates in detail, but it would be foolish to imagine that they were not affected.

What's more, the researchers found striking disparities in the speed with which different teams learned. All teams came from highly respected institutions with experience in adopting innovations and received the same three-day training session. Yet, in the course of 50 cases, some teams managed to halve their operating time while others improved hardly at all. Practice, it turned out, did not necessarily make perfect. The crucial variable was *how* the surgeons and their teams practiced.

Richard Bohmer, the only physician among the Harvard researchers, made several visits to observe one of the quickest-learning teams and one of the slowest, and he was startled by the contrast. The surgeon on the fast-learning team was actually quite inexperienced compared with the one on the slow-learning team. But he made sure to pick team members with whom he had worked well before and to keep them together through the first 15 cases before allowing any new members. He had the team go through a dry run before the first case, then deliberately scheduled six operations in the first week, so little would be forgotten in between. He convened the team before each case to discuss it in detail and afterward to debrief. He made sure results were tracked carefully. And Bohmer noticed that the surgeon was not the stereotypical Napoleon with a knife. Unbidden, he told Bohmer, "The surgeon needs to be willing to allow himself to become a partner [with the rest of the team] so he can accept input." At the other hospital, by contrast, the surgeon chose his operating team almost randomly and did not keep it together. In the first seven cases, the team had different members every time, which is to say that it was no team at all. And the surgeon had no pre-briefings, no debriefings, no tracking of ongoing results.

The Harvard Business School study offered some hopeful news. We can do things that have a dramatic effect on our rate of improvement—like being more deliberate about how we train, and about tracking progress, whether with students and residents or with senior surgeons and nurses. But the study's other implications are less reassuring. No matter how accomplished, surgeons trying something new got worse before they got better, and the learning curve proved longer, and was affected by a far more complicated range of factors, than anyone had realized.

This, I suspect, is the reason for the physician's dodge: the "I just assist" rap; the "We have a new procedure for this that you are perfect for" speech; the "You need a central line" without the "I am still learning how to do this." Sometimes we do feel obliged to admit when we're doing something for the first time, but even then we tend to quote the published complication rates of experienced surgeons. Do we ever tell patients that, because we are still new at something, their risks will inevitably be higher, and that they'd likely do better with doctors who are more experienced? Do we ever say that we need them to agree to it anyway? I've never seen it. Given the stakes, who in his right mind would agree to be practiced upon?

Many dispute this presumption: "Look, most people understand what it is to be a doctor," a health policy expert insisted, when I visited him in his office not long ago. "We have to stop lying to our patients. Can people take on choices for societal benefit?" He paused and then answered his question. "Yes," he said firmly.

It would certainly be a graceful and happy solution. We'd ask patients— honestly, openly—and they'd say yes. Hard to imagine, though. I noticed on the expert's desk a picture of his child, born just a few months before, and a completely unfair question popped into my mind. "So did you let the resident deliver?" I asked.

There was silence for a moment. "No," he admitted. "We didn't even allow residents in the room."

One reason I doubt whether we could sustain a system of medical training that depended on people saying "Yes, you can practice on me" is that I myself have said no. When my eldest child, Walker, was eleven days old, he suddenly went into congestive heart failure from what proved to be a severe cardiac defect. His aorta was not transposed, but a long segment of it had failed to grow at all. My wife and I were beside ourselves with fear— his kidneys and liver began failing, too—but he made it to surgery, the repair was a success, and although his recovery was erratic, after two and a half weeks he was ready to come home.

We were by no means in the clear, however. He was born a healthy six pounds plus but now, a month old, he weighed only five, and would need strict monitoring to insure that he gained weight. He was on two cardiac medications from which he would have to be weaned. And in the longer term, the doctors warned us, his repair would prove inadequate. As Walker grew, his aorta would require either dilation with a balloon or replacement by surgery. They could not say precisely when and how many such procedures would be necessary over the years. A pediatric cardiologist would have to follow him closely and decide.

Walker was about to be discharged, and we had not indicated who that cardiologist would be. In the hospital, he had been cared for by a full team of cardiologists, ranging from fellows in specialty training to attendings who had practiced for decades. The day before we took Walker home, one of the young fellows approached me, offering his card and suggesting a time to bring Walker to see him. Of those on the team, he had put in the most time caring for Walker. He saw Walker when we brought him in inexplicably short of breath, made the diagnosis, got Walker the drugs that stabilized him, coordinated with the surgeons, and came to see us twice a day to answer our questions. Moreover, I knew, this was how fellows always got their patients. Most families don't know the subtle gradations among players, and after a team has saved their child's life they take whatever appointment they're handed.

But I knew the differences. "I'm afraid we're thinking of seeing Dr. Newburger," I said. She was the hospital's associate cardiologist-in-chief, and a published expert on conditions like Walker's. The young physician looked crestfallen. It was nothing against him, I said. She just had more experience, that was all.

"You know, there is always an attending backing me up," he said. I shook my head.

I know this was not fair. My son had an unusual problem. The fellow needed the experience. As a resident, I of all people should have understood this. But I was not torn about the decision. This was my child. Given a choice, I will always choose the best care I can for him. How can anybody be expected to do otherwise? Certainly, the future of medicine should not rely on it.

In a sense, then, the physician's dodge is inevitable. Learning must be stolen, taken as a kind of bodily eminent domain. And it was, during Walker's stay—on many occasions, now that I think back on it. A resident intubated him. A surgical trainee scrubbed in for his operation. The cardiology fellow put in one of his central lines. If I had the option to have someone more experienced, I would have taken it. But this was simply how the system worked—no such choices were offered—and so I went along.

The advantage of this coldhearted machinery is not merely that it gets the learning done. If learning is necessary but causes harm, then above all it ought to apply to everyone alike. Given a choice, people wriggle out, and such choices are not offered equally. They belong to the connected and the knowledgeable, to insiders over outsiders, to the doctor's child but not the truck driver's. If everyone cannot have a choice, maybe it is better if no one can.

It is 2 P.M. I am in the intensive-care unit. A nurse tells me Mr. G.'s central line has clotted off. Mr. G. has been in the hospital for more than a month now. He is in his late sixties, from South Boston, emaciated, exhausted, holding on by a thread—or a line, to be precise. He has several holes in his small bowel, and the bilious contents leak out onto his skin through two small reddened openings in the concavity of his abdomen. His only chance is to be fed by vein and wait for these fistulae to heal. He needs a new central line.

I could do it, I suppose. I am the experienced one now. But experience brings a new role: I am expected to teach the procedure instead. "See one, do one, teach one," the saying goes, and it is only half in jest.

There is a junior resident on the service. She has done only one or two lines before. I tell her about Mr. G. I ask her if she is free to do a new line. She misinterprets this as a question. She says she still has patients to see and a case coming up later. Could I do the line? I tell her no. She is unable to hide a grimace. She is burdened, as I was burdened, and perhaps frightened, as I was frightened.

She begins to focus when I make her talk through the steps—a kind of dry run, I figure. She hits nearly all the steps, but forgets about checking the labs and about Mr. G.'s nasty allergy to heparin, which is in the flush for the line. I make sure she registers this, then tell her to get set up and page me.

I am still adjusting to this role. It is painful enough taking responsibility for one's own failures. Being handmaiden to another's is something else entirely. It occurs to me that I could have broken open a kit and had her do an actual dry run. Then again maybe I can't. The kits must cost a couple of hundred dollars each. I'll have to find out for the next time.

Half an hour later, I get the page. The patient is draped. The resident is in her gown and gloves. She tells me that she has saline to flush the line with and that his labs are fine.

"Have you got the towel roll?" I ask.

She forgot the towel roll. I roll up a towel and slip it beneath Mr. G.'s back. I ask him if he's all right. He nods. After all he's been through, there is only resignation in his eyes.

The junior resident picks out a spot for the stick. The patient is hauntingly thin. I see every rib and fear that the resident will puncture his lung. She injects the numbing medication. Then she puts the big needle in, and the angle looks all wrong. I motion for her to reposition. This only makes her more uncertain. She pushes in deeper and I know she does not have it. She draws back on the syringe: no blood. She takes out the needle and tries again. And again the angle looks wrong. This time, Mr. G. feels the jab and jerks up in pain. I hold his arm. She gives him more numbing medication. It is all I can do not to take over. But she cannot learn without doing, I tell myself. I decide to let her have one more try.

## Case Study:
## The "Student Doctor" and a Wary Patient
Marc D. Basson, Gerald Dworkin,
and Eric J. Cassell

Like many medical schools, State Medical College permits its third-year students to rotate through Anesthesiology for a month. During the first week, students follow Anesthesiology residents as they visit patients. Then students are assigned their own patients. After obtaining informed consent, they administer anesthesia under supervision.

James Denton is one such third-year student, rotating through the Smithville VA, an affiliated hospital. His first solo patient is Robert Criswell, a sixty-four-year-old man with metastatic prostate cancer who is scheduled to undergo bilateral orchiectomy (castration) in the morning. Criswell has a history of heavy smoking and poor pulmonary function, so James reasons that a spinal anesthetic would be safer than general anesthesia.

The attending anesthesiologist tentatively agrees to this plan. "You've done lumbar punctures before, haven't you?" the anesthesiologist asks. James says that he has done one spinal tap previously, but had great difficulty with it. He adds that he has seen three others performed. "Well, you've got to learn some time," responds the anesthesiologist. "Don't worry, I'll be with you."

James returns to the ward and finds Mr. Criswell. The residents have advised him to introduce himself as "Doctor" Denton so as not to frighten the patient unnecessarily. Some of James's fellow students use deliberately ambiguous phrases such as "one of the anesthesiology team that will be taking care of you." James selects a popular alternative, introducing himself as "a student doctor from Anesthesiology."

Marc D. Basson, Gerald Dworkin, and Eric J. Cassell, "Case Study: The 'Student Doctor' and a Wary Patient," from *The Hastings Center Report*, vol. 12, 27–28. © 1982. Reprinted by permission of The Hastings Center and M. Basson.

James tells Mr. Criswell that he would like to use spinal anesthesia and explains the procedure for lumbar puncture. "You should know," he says as he fills in the consent sheet, "that like any other medical procedure a lumbar puncture has risks, including bleeding, infection, paralysis, pain, and perhaps even death. Also, a few people develop severe headaches after such a procedure and we will ask you to lie flat for twenty-four hours afterwards to lessen the chances of this happening."

"Tell me, doctor," Criswell asks, "have you ever had any of these problems with your patients?" James feels uneasy at being called a doctor and at Criswell's assumption that he has done many lumbar punctures before, but he decides that this is not the time to bring up his inexperience. "No, never, although I have seen one moderately severe spinal headache lasting for three days in a friend's patient," he responds.

"That's OK, I can take a headache," Criswell says as he signs the consent form. "I didn't want to insult you or anything. It's just that I've heard all kinds of stories about those medical students from the university coming over here to practice on the vets and leaving them paralyzed for life."

How should James Denton introduce himself? Is he morally or legally obligated to discuss his inexperience in obtaining an informed consent? Would it make a difference if the patient had never raised the issue of experience?

*Marc D. Basson*

**Commentary**

Gerald Dworkin

Considering the frequency with which situations similar to the one described in this case arise in everyday medical practice, it is surprising that the legitimacy of what occurs has not occasioned greater ethical scrutiny. Perhaps this is a specific instance of the generalization that the amount of attention paid to ethical issues is inversely proportional to their frequency in practice. Abortions performed because the life of the mother is threatened by pregnancy account for a minuscule proportion of the total, but occupy a fairly high proportion of the philosophical literature. This case, involving the training of students by allowing them to practice technical procedures on patients under supervision, occurs routinely. Yet the only public discussion I have seen concerned the bizarre case of a salesman from a medical instrumentation company who was allowed to operate on patients—without their knowledge—in order to demonstrate the nature and value of his company's products.

We are not faced here with a moral dilemma. This is not a situation in which there are good reasons of a fairly weighty nature for and against a certain course of action. A patient is being misled as to the qualifications, experience, and competence of his "healer." He thinks that James is a doctor (when he is not). He thinks that James has performed this procedure many times before (when he has not). He thinks that James has fairly wide experience with the possible side effects of the procedures (when he has not). While the violation of informed consent is not as gross as that which occurs very commonly when a surgeon does not tell his patient that the operation will actually be performed by a resident or intern (under the surgeon's supervision), the interference with the patient's ability to make an informed choice is clear. In the absence of exceptions to the principle of informed consent, we must condemn this practice.

By exceptions to the principle of informed consent, I mean factors such as impossibility (the patient is unconscious or an infant), waiver (the patient has waived the right to be informed), external justification (getting the consent of the patient would violate more important rights of others), internal justification (the ends served by the rule would be better served by making an exception).

In this case I do not see that such factors are present, and I conclude therefore that James ought to inform his patient of his status, experience, and qualifications. The patient then could either decide to go ahead or ask for a more experienced physician. The fact that the patient has explicitly raised the issue of experience is only relevant insofar as it offers empirical evidence that this patient is particularly worried about this matter. But it is reasonable to assume that all patients have a concern about their doctor's experience and competence, and would want to know that this is the first time he or she is performing a fairly risky procedure.

This answer to the particular issue does not, however, address the more general concern underlying the practice; namely, that we would all be worse off if surgeons and anesthesiologists could not be trained and training requires "hands-on" experience. The solution is not deception, but finding ways to make it attractive for patients to agree to being the subjects of such training. It is reasonable for teaching hospitals to claim that the quality of care they provide is better than that of nonteaching hospitals, and that the "price" for this is that patients agree to being part of the training process. As long as this is done forthrightly, and patients have some degree of choice as to the hospitals they enter, I see no objection. Or perhaps there could be a price differential, depending on whether a doctor performed the operation or merely supervised it. This is common practice for analysts-in-training, who charge their patients a greatly reduced fee.

It is worth noting that the problem of "hands-on" training is not confined to the medical profession. Airline pilots, automobile mechanics, sushi chefs, student drivers, hairdressers, psychotherapists—all have to impose risks on others in order to learn their skills. But those who bear the risks ought to be aware that they are doing so and be compensated in some fashion for their cooperation.

### Commentary

Eric J. Cassell

This case raises two distinct questions. The first is how the medical student, James Denton, should respond to the patient who questions his qualifications. The second is the more general question of whether medical educators are justified in allowing trainees to have primary responsibility for the care of the sick when more qualified physicians are available.

James Denton is obligated to tell the patient, Robert Criswell, the truth. But that is not the end of the matter, it is merely the beginning. Ethical issues such as truth-telling are too often dealt with as though they stood alone and timeless, like public monuments. These problems achieve their importance because of their place in human relations—of persons to themselves and to others. In medical practice, telling the truth serves something larger than itself. It is, for example, an important aspect of trust, and trust is fundamental in the doctor-patient relationship. But trust is a complex, poorly understood matter and so it is easier to discuss truth-telling in the same oversimplified way that we often discuss other ethical issues like autonomy.

Consider this case again. Robert Criswell has metastatic cancer of the prostate and he is about to have his testicles removed. From this history we do not know much about him, but if he is like most of us, he may be frightened by his situation. He is in a VA hospital where the care is sometimes impersonal and where his need for reassurance and for the information that might reduce his uncertainties may not be met.

Into that setting walks James Denton, third-year student cum anesthesiologist, also frightened and unsure. The way this case history is recounted suggests that they are adversaries. On the contrary, they are natural allies (like many, perhaps most, doctors and sick patients) because they need each other. Should Denton be honest? Of course he must tell the truth. But then he must actively set out to win Criswell's trust because both he and the patient need it. He must make it clear that he is a novice, but just because of that he will be more attentive and more concerned about Criswell's well-being than another, more experienced anesthesiologist might be. For this and other reasons (including the fact that information can itself be therapeutic when properly employed) he will carefully explain what is to be done, why it is being done, and what it means to Criswell, answering each of the patient's questions (and getting the correct information when he does not know). He will point out that the attending physician will be watching over them to make sure nothing goes wrong, and that he, James Denton, will visit Criswell while he is in the hospital.

For the rest of his life, if he takes care of patients, James Denton will be talking people into doing things that, while for their benefit, may be fraught with risk and fear. And on many of those occasions he will be pursued by doubts and well aware that others might do things better. That is the nature of medical care. Of course, when trust has been created and nurtured, it must not be betrayed because that is worse than lying.

This case does not describe an isolated instance, although "see one, do one, teach one" is an exaggeration of the problem. It is the strength of American medical education that physicians learn while taking care of patients under the guidance of more experienced teachers. However, the teachers, especially attending physicians, could often give better, more efficient, and less costly care to a particular patient than their trainees. Indeed, the student or house officer may be learning on someone who has been the patient of the teacher for many years. In that case the attending physician further helps the doctor in training by including him or her within the bonds of trust that have developed over those years. How, then, can we justify this method of education? Without this system of supervised learning by doing, teachers themselves would not be well trained and the qualifications of the whole profession would suffer.

What I have touched on so briefly describes a complex system of relationships and bonds that are part of the moral nature of the institution of medicine. Many would be quick to point out the ethical error if James Denton lied to Robert Criswell about his professional status. Those same critics, both inside and outside of the profession, might consider it old-fashioned, "hierarchical," or too conservative to worry about such important moral flaws as the failure to give deference to attending physicians and patients, the failure to protect the bonds of trust between patient and doctor, and the failure to protect both the past and the future of the profession of medicine. But a lie by James Denton threatens only Denton and Criswell, while those other "old-fashioned" flaws endanger the integrity of the profession, without which no one would take this case seriously.

## A Student's View of a
## Medical Teaching Exercise
Abenaa Brewster

Physicians are usually careful to explain the purpose and format of a teaching session when asking a patient to take part. Failure to do so when the patient is poorly educated or of a different cultural background may seriously disturb the patient and mislead the other participants. Consider the events at a recent neurology conference at a Boston teaching hospital.

The resident began by describing the case of "a 52-year-old postmenopausal black woman with a history of breast cancer at age 46 treated by mastectomy and radiation." She went on to say:

> A year ago the patient had back and leg pain and was found to have diffuse skeletal metastases. She was treated with local radiation and tamoxifen, with moderate relief. The sudden onset of excruciating pain in her right thigh 48 hours ago led to hospitalization. Because of some memory loss and apparent confusion, she was seen by a consulting neurologist, who suggested that she might have cerebral metastases. Her mental status is intact, but she has some difficulty remembering names.

The patient was brought into the room in a wheelchair, accompanied by her daughter and sister. The attending neurologist pulled his chair close to the patient and asked where she was from. She replied in a thick Southern accent that she was from a small town in Arkansas, and she introduced her relatives. She was then asked whether she recognized anyone in the room, to name someone, and to point to those whom she could not name. She seemed bewildered by the request. The conference continued as follows:

Abenaa Brewster, "A Student's View of a Medical Teaching Exercise," from *New England Journal of Medicine*, vol. 329, 1971–1972. © 1993 by the Massachusetts Medical Society. Reprinted by permission of the publisher.

Neurologist: How old were you when you had the operation on your breast, and what has happened since?

Patient: Honey, I was maybe 46, but I can't remember all the things from back then that you want me to remember. I want to see the doctor who operated on me, honey. That's who I want to talk to.

Neurologist: What's that about money?

He turned to the room.

Neurologist: What is she saying about money?

Resident: She's calling you "honey."

Everyone in the room laughed, and the neurologist appeared embarrassed.

Patient: I'm not trying to pick you up or nothing, I'm just calling you "honey"; it's just a saying.

Neurologist: Can you try to raise your leg, please.

He leaned forward to hold her leg.

Patient: Don't touch me. Everybody wants me to raise this and raise that. I can't do anything with the leg. Don't ask me to do anything. I'm not doing anything. I'm a smart woman, you know; I'm not stupid. Y'all think that I'm stupid. I don't know anything about those pictures over there [pointing to the X-ray films], but I'm a smart woman, very smart.

The patient started to cry.

Neurologist: It must be very difficult trying to cope with your problems. We will all try to come up with some suitable treatment to help you.

He signaled to the resident that the session was over.

Patient: I know that y'all gonna laugh when I leave, oooh Lord. Y'all gonna laugh, oooh Lord.

The patient was wheeled out of the room as a few people said goodbye.

Neurologist: Well, that was *something.* She is obviously volatile and disinhibited, which probably reflects metastases to her frontal lobes. I thought it best not to persist, for she was obviously being very uncooperative.

A discussion about the patient's medical condition ensued, during which a radiologist indicated that he saw no evidence of brain metastases.

From the beginning of the encounter between the attending neurologist and the patient, a mismatch of agendas was evident. Had time and care been taken at the outset, an agenda could have been set to benefit both parties. The neurologist's goals were to seek additional information about the patient's medical history, to determine her mental status, and to clarify the nature of any neurologic deficits. A further objective might have been to demonstrate to the residents and students a method for establishing a sound patient-doctor relationship.

The patient, for whatever reason, assumed she was to see the doctor who had operated on her years before. Her goal was surely not to be embarrassed for calling a doctor "honey" and not to feel humiliated because she could not recognize faces in the crowd. Similarly, she did not understand why she was asked to answer questions that had been asked several times before, nor why a doctor she had not previously met wished to examine her in front of strangers and to display her lack of motor function.

I could not help but feel that had the patient been a well-educated woman speaking standard English, the demonstration would have been very different. Before the conference, the resident would have explained to the patient what she could expect. During the meeting, the attending neurologist would probably have told her why he was asking her to identify people in the room. And had these simple amenities not been observed, the discussion after her departure might have focused on why she had not been properly informed. The resident would have been asked whether she had forgotten to explain to the patient that questions would be asked and a neurologic examination carried out for the benefit of physicians who had not had the opportunity to read her chart.

Furthermore, I believe that if there had been even one nonwhite doctor in that room, adjectives like "volatile" and "disinhibited" might not have been used so readily. Indeed, an appreciation for the patient's frankness might have replaced "disinhibited," and admiration of her pride and her effort to control her life might have replaced "volatile."

When faced with people who differ from ourselves, or with "difficult" patients, an easy way out is to seek a medical label for behavior that we cannot understand or control. How often do we base differential diagnoses on stereotypes?

Such attitudes and actions on the part of physicians can impede the discovery of nonmedical explanations for what often proves to be, after all, normal behavior. They put us at risk of depriving patients of opportunities to contribute to their own medical care and prevent us from caring properly for people whom we do not understand. They can stifle opportunities to learn more about people of other races, classes, or cultural backgrounds. Finally, they deflect us from giving all our patients unconditional respect.

**Note**

I am indebted to Dr. Howard Hiatt for his advice and support.

# *Primum non tacere*:
# An Ethics of Speaking Up
James Dwyer

During the last five years I have conducted ethics courses, seminars, and case conferences for medical students. I have also had many informal discussions with students at all stages of their medical training. Yet I am still surprised by how many students know and refer to the Hippocratic maxim to do no harm. Some even cite the Latin version: *Primum non nocere*. I wish, however, that more medical students would also keep in mind a Socratic maxim: *Primum non tacere*. First, do not be silent.

When I encourage students to articulate ethical issues that they face as students, they often describe situations where they must decide whether to speak up or keep quiet. The following are cases that students have described and that I have altered somewhat and then formulated from a student's perspective.

  *1. Spos* (acronym for "subhuman piece of shit").[1] Before I entered medical school I read *House of God*, but I didn't find it very amusing. I was troubled by the attitudes the characters displayed, and I told myself that I would try to be more respectful of patients. I assumed that speaking about patients in derogatory terms was a fad that would be over by the time I began my clerkships at the hospital. That was not the case. During my first rotation my resident presented me with a new admission: "Here's your patient. He's a 40-year-old Hispanic male, a shooter, a real spos."

  I wondered whether I should say anything. I didn't like that language and the attitude it displayed, but it wasn't my job to train the house staff. On the other hand, if I didn't say anything, I'd seem to accept the judgments and attitudes I want to avoid.

  *2. Informed Consent.*[2] I always thought that informed consent was inte-

James Dwyer, "Primum non tacere: An Ethics of Speaking Up," from *The Hastings Center Report*, vol. 24, 13–18. © 1994. Reprinted by permission of The Hastings Center.

gral to the doctor-patient relationship, that it was really one aspect of good communication with patients. Yet some people view it differently, as a bureaucratic hassle imposed by people outside medicine. This difference became painfully clear during my first week in the clerkship. My resident told me to "consent" one of his patients. This was my second day. I had never met the patient and had no idea what the risks of the proposed procedure were. So I politely asked my resident about the risks, but he told me with a slight sense of annoyance that the patient will sign anything. What were my choices? I could say something to the resident. I could just get the signature. I could look up the procedure in a textbook. Or I could ask someone who might explain the procedure to me. In fact, I asked another resident who told me a bit about the procedure.

An hour later my resident saw me again and said that the team had decided to include a second procedure. He told me to simply write the second procedure onto the form and to use the same pen. I didn't want to be party to this sham, but I also didn't want to jeopardize my grade.

3. *Practice Makes Perfect.*[3] I understand that this hospital is a teaching hospital and that students, residents, and fellows are here to learn. The fact that we learn on patients means that some patients are subjected to additional pain, inconvenience, and physical examinations. I guess there's a kind of bargain: we learn medicine on people who are mostly poor, and they get care they might not otherwise have access to. Whether or not this arrangement is fair, I've come to accept it. But I never imagined that people would practice a procedure that wasn't medically indicated.

Late one night I was working with a resident in the labor and delivery room. The patient was in labor, and the resident decided to do a forceps delivery. I didn't see the indication. The woman didn't seem very fatigued, and there were no apparent complications. I didn't know the exact statistics, but I was sure that a forceps delivery involved some risk to the fetus. I didn't know what to do. If I asked what the indications were, the resident was sure to have some rationalization. If I told an attending physician the next day, I'd create a lot of trouble and no good would come of it. If I did nothing, I'd feel ashamed—I went into medicine to help people.

4. *An Important Finding.*[4] One of the patients I was following was Mr. Z, a 52-year-old diabetic man with bedsores. After rounds it was my job to dress his wounds. As I was helping him turn over in bed, my hand pressed against his left side. I felt a crackling under his skin. "Like rice crispies under the skin," I remembered the lecturer telling us two years ago. I knew what that meant: crepitus, a sign of infection by a gas-producing organism.

Since I was pretty sure, I told the intern about my finding. I was polite, but direct. I told him that I thought the patient had crepitus and that he should take a look.

I asked about Mr. Z when I saw the intern that afternoon. He said that Mr. Z didn't have crepitus and that we would check on him in the morning. Before I went home that evening I stopped by to see Mr. Z again. His general condition seemed worse. I pressed on his side again and felt the same crackling. I wondered whether I should speak to the intern again that evening, go talk to the senior resident, or just go home.

5. *What Were We Doing?*[5] One of the first patients I had in pediatrics was a two-year-old child dying of AIDS. What bothered me most about the case was what we were doing to the child. It seemed like we were always drawing blood or doing something to it. Once we did two lumbar punctures in one day!

After a while I understood the technical reasons for each test and procedure we did, but I didn't really understand the overall strategy. I wondered what all our treatment would accomplish for the child. So I spoke to my resident. I told her I was troubled by the pain we were inflicting and asked whether she thought the child would recover enough to go home. She didn't think the child would live much longer, and she too was troubled by the aggressive treatment that the attending physician ordered. The attending wanted to do everything possible, and no one was going to fault him for doing too much.

I felt I should cautiously broach my concern with the attending physician, but I saw clearly that the resident was unwilling to say anything to him.

### Keeping Quiet

The ethical issue I want to discuss is whether students should voice their disagreement in situations like these. I will begin by considering the view that the best course of action for students is to keep quiet.

Melvin Konner describes how, as a medical student, he came to adopt the practice of keeping quiet.[6] His first clinical rotation was an assignment in one of the units of the hospital. At the beginning of the rotation the director of the unit explained some alphabet soup: clinical reminders formulated as a series of letters or acronyms. Konner asked a question that he thought was relevant and important. The curt response convinced him that he was making a mistake. At that point he says: "I reminded myself of some of my own alphabet soup. . . . *k.m.s., you jerk,* I said to myself, as loudly as I could inside my head. *keep mouth shut. At least until you get the lay of the land. Or until you have something indispensable to say"* (p. 55).

Just after this reminder Konner noticed that a patient who looked to be in pain had appeared in the waiting room. Although the other staff seemed not to have noticed the patient, Konner kept quiet. But after a while the thought that the patient might need attention prompted him to say something. The director chastised him for interrupting. Konner reflects:

> It was the last message I needed to get from him. k.m.s. was from then on not only easy but second nature to me. I faded into the woodwork in every situation. I rarely if ever spoke unless I had been directly addressed. This is the army, I thought. Every time you open your mouth you create complications for yourself. It was a rule I followed throughout the rest of my medical training; making exceptions only when I was in the presence of the unusual medical teacher who was not overbearingly arrogant, and whom I instinctively felt I could trust. (p. 57)

Thus keeping quiet became the practice that Konner tried to adhere to during the course of medical school.

On a number of occasions Konner stifled questions that he wanted to ask. Once he had a question about the way morning rounds were conducted, but he said to himself: "Mine was not to reason why, and I followed faithfully and quietly, suppressing even the most seemingly pertinent questions about treatment and course of illness" (p. 93). On another occasion he wondered why a patient did not have DNR (do not resuscitate) status, but he said nothing. Often he reflected on the nonphysical aspects of healing, but he kept quiet about his reflections. When a young woman with cancer died on the wards, he thought about the case: "As much as I wanted to hear some discussion about it—even a strictly medical discussion would have been better than nothing—I had developed sense enough not to ask. My concerns, I realized, were idiosyncratic. Nobody wanted to hear about them, not even most of my fellow students. I could simplify my life best by keeping them to myself, and I certainly wanted to simplify my life" (p. 294). Thus Konner came to believe that most of his questions were unwelcome complications.

Although the practice of keeping quiet may simplify one's life, it is morally problematic in at least two ways. When keeping quiet is adopted as a blanket policy, it covers up important differences between cases. Keeping quiet about improper care, for example, is importantly different from keeping quiet about one's beliefs about the spiritual aspects of healing. Also, when keeping quiet is proposed as a strategy for getting through medical school, it simply ignores the ethical question of whether students have some obligation to speak up. What is needed is a discussion of the ethics of speaking up.

### Students' Obligations

Speaking up may subject students to various risks and repercussions. They may be graded by someone they have offended by speaking up; they may be ridiculed for asking a question or voicing their concerns; they may be seen as a lone dissenter or even a disloyal team member; they may be viewed as unprofessional for criticizing other professionals; and, if they go over someone's head, they may be seen as rats or tattletales. These possibilities are not trivial: how students are viewed by others can affect their career prospects as well as their sense of themselves.

Since speaking up places students at some risk, this kind of engagement requires a degree of courage. A need for courage is not limited to the situations depicted at the beginning of this essay, but is common to learning and practicing medicine. Students face a risk of infection from HIV, HBV, tuberculosis, and other diseases. Yet for the most part they draw blood or do what needs to be done, in spite of the risk to themselves. Many students, however, who act courageously in the face of contagious disease hesitate to speak up. They see procedures like drawing blood as part of what a good physician has to do, but view speaking up as an individual choice that goes beyond the practice of medicine. I do not share this view. Especially now, when medicine is often practiced in large institutions with a number of people involved in the care of an individual patient, speaking up is something physicians may have to do to meet their responsibilities to patients, colleagues, and the profession of medicine.

It is up to the medical profession to set standards of care and to regulate its members. This crucial task is one of the characteristics of professional life. Neither society as a whole nor patients individually are well positioned to take over this work. Patients, especially, rarely see and know enough to set standards and to judge who falls short. Thus physicians are entrusted with a moral and legal responsibility to assess their colleagues and to report those who are incompetent or unethical.[7] But their moral commitment goes beyond a duty to establish review boards and to report flagrant cases. Patients also entrust physicians to engage their colleagues and institutions about less flagrant, more everyday matters. This engagement might often take the form of questions and discussions. Even in cases where reasonable physicians may disagree, physicians may have a duty to do just that: to voice their disagreement and to question the reasoning of others.

But just because full-fledged physicians have an obligation to speak up, it does not follow that medical students do. Students are not professionals and have much less power and authority than practicing physicians. They may therefore have fewer or different obligations. At a minimum, students are obligated to take notice of bad practices and to try to conduct themselves in a better way when they become full-fledged physicians. But is learning from bad examples enough? Might students be obligated to engage themselves in a more active way?

Students, like all human beings, have a moral obligation to prevent serious harm when they can do so at little risk or cost to themselves. We can think of this obligation as a natural duty—independent of promises, contracts, and roles.[8] There are, however, problems with appealing to a natural duty in this context. Students face many situations where the duty does not apply because the potential harm to the patient is not grave and the risks of speaking up are significant. Furthermore, since a natural duty is (by definition) an obligation that every human being has, it does not specify what obligations students have in virtue of their role as medical students.

To determine what specific obligations medical students have, it is helpful to clarify what their role is. Medical students often assume different roles during different stages of training, in different departments, at different clinics and hospitals, and with different residents and attending physicians. They act as observers, auxiliaries for residents, caregivers, counselors, patient advocates, researchers, and even teachers. Yet their primary role, function, and purpose is to learn to be good physicians. The obligations implicit in this role are the ones that need to be elaborated.

It is the work of medical students to acquire the knowledge, skills, and habits that good physicians need. To acquire these skills and habits, and even this knowledge, it is not enough for students passively to observe medical practice and to note what they will do when they are full-fledged physicians. They must practice things now—take medical histories, do physical exams, start ivs, make differential diagnoses—to have the skills and habits they will need to do a good job when they are practicing physicians. Among the skills and habits that students need to practice are those that good physicians call upon in ethically problematic situations. Students must act now to develop habits they will need later.

The key concept here is the idea of habit. Any conduct as complex as the practice of medicine depends on more than abstract knowledge, viewed as a fund of facts and theories. Such conduct also depends on habits, acquired but not always conscious ways of action and perception.[9] One of the reasons that habits are important is that they are like resources or skills that can be called into use when needed. When students are faced with situations like the ones depicted at the beginning of this essay, they have an opportunity to develop habits that are important for the good practice of medicine. It might be nice if such situations never arose—just as it might be nice if there were never any cases of tuberculosis—but such situations do arise, and students must learn to deal with them. If students do not engage themselves in these situations, they fail to develop and exercise the qualities of a good physician. It is not enough to observe these situations now and to vow to act if similar situations arise after full professional status has been attained. Habits of reflection, character, and intervention need to be developed and exercised if they are to be ready at hand in the future.

### Learning and Caring

What I have said so far may seem to overemphasize the idea of learning at the expense of the idea of caring. I can imagine someone formulating the following objection: "Keeping quiet in situations like the ones depicted is more than a failure to seize an opportunity to develop important skills. It is not a failure of learning but of caring. In fact, keeping quiet is a failure to act as a caring physician." As a way of responding to this objection, I want to explain how a failure to speak up in certain situations is a failure of learning and caring.

The first thing I want to say about the complex relationship between learning and caring concerns the connection between habit and character. Acquiring a habit is often more than developing an isolated skill that can be called upon when needed. The acquisition of a habit often amounts to the formation or alteration of a part of character. It is true that habits are like resources or skills that can be called into use when needed. But habits have another important feature. They act like elements of character that influence or color conduct even when they are not in overt use. Habits are not only ready at hand; they are always at work.

John Dewey notes this feature when he remarks that habits are "operative in some subdued form even when not obviously dominating activity" (p. 39). And he gives a convincing example:

> The habit of walking is expressed in what a man sees when he keeps still, even in dreams. The recognition of distances and directions of things from his place at rest is the obvious proof of this statement. The habit of locomotion is latent in the sense that it is covered up, counteracted, by a habit of seeing which is definitely at the fore. But counteraction is not suppression. . . . Everything that a man who has the habit of locomotion does and thinks, he does and thinks differently on that account. (pp. 36–37)

In this way certain habits may influence conduct even when these habits are not called into direct use.

Because many habits influence perception and conduct even when they are not dominant in a particular activity, these habits amount to or are connected with traits of character. The kinds of habits needed in situations like the ones depicted are not isolated skills that are separate from the character of a caring physician. Rather, there is a positive connection between these habits and the character traits of a caring physician. Yet it would be somewhat misleading to say that students need to act in those situations so that they will learn to be caring physicians. It is more accurate to say that they need to act in those situations so that they will not learn to be uncaring physicians. I'll explain why I put the matter that way.

There is, of course, a relationship between caring and learning to fulfill one's obligations and responsibilities. I want to suggest an account of this relationship in the experience of medical students. Some accounts of ethical obligation start with rational egoists and show how they acquire and come to feel that they have obligations to others. In these accounts obligations arise to fill a vacant space—a space where previously there was no felt moral concern. Whatever the merits of these accounts, as either moral theories or theories of moral development, they do not capture the place and function of specific obligations in the moral life of medical students.

For the most part, medical students are committed and feel committed to caring about and for patients. They begin their training with a felt sense of moral concern, and then they learn specific obligations and responsibilities. Instead of thinking of students as coming to have and perceive obligations where they previously felt no commitment or moral concern, it is more accurate to think of learning specific obligations as a process that directs or even limits students' diffuse sense of moral concern. What students learn is to clarify and define their obligations and responsibilities to patients and others. This learning may only be successful when there is a background of moral concern.

There are two dangers in this learning process. If responsibilities are not clarified and delineated, students' moral concern will remain diffuse and probably ineffective. It seems to demand everything and to point in no direction. The second danger is the more common one in professional training. If responsibilities are defined too narrowly, technically, or legalistically, there is a danger that moral concern and imagination will be lost.[10] The danger is that very narrowly defined responsibilities and obligations will be substituted for a sense of moral concern that was somewhat open-ended, searching, and imaginative. When the sense of moral concern is fixed on and exhausted by the technical responsibilities that have been learned, the result is a competent technician with a narrow sense of professional responsibility.

If medical students learn to keep quiet in all situations, and do so without qualms, then their sense of moral concern is exhausted by some narrow account of responsibilities and obligations. If they experience qualms but still keep quiet, then their sense of moral concern exceeds the narrow account but has not found expression at a cost that is acceptable to them. Thus it is true that the practice of always keeping quiet is a failure of caring. It is a failure in the process of learning to care, a failure that occurs either by allowing narrowly defined responsibilities to exhaust a sense of caring or by not adequately expressing a residual, open-ended sense of caring.

### When and How

To further their development as caring physicians, students need to consider exactly when and how they should speak up. Although these considerations depend very much on the particular situations, there are some general factors to keep in mind. In trying to decide whether to speak up in a particular case, students should consider the nature and certainty of their judgment, their specific role in the situation, the potential harm to patients, the probable effectiveness of speaking up, and the likely cost to themselves if they do speak up. I'll say a few words about each of these points.

Students may be unsure of their judgments in two different ways. They may not have enough experience to know with certainty whether a particular course of action is medically appropriate, or they may have doubts about their own ethical judgment in a particular situation. Yet the existence of either kind of uncertainty is not necessarily a reason for keeping quiet, since there is usually some degree of uncertainty in medicine and ethics. Students need to find the appropriate threshold of certainty for voicing their concerns. This threshold may depend on a number of the factors mentioned.

Variations in students' specific roles make an ethical difference. When students are actively engaged in patient care, they have a greater obligation to speak up about situations that involve their patients, whereas in situations they merely hear about because they are on the wards their obligation is correspondingly less. Of course, if the matter is serious enough, they should speak up even if they stand on the periphery of the situation.

Obviously, the potential harm to the patient is a very important factor. When there is a serious threat to the patient's well-being, students should speak up even if they are somewhat uncertain and somewhat on the periphery. They should speak up, for example, in cases where they make important findings, believe certain tests should be done, or think that the proposed courses of action involve serious and unjustified risks. When the potential harm to the patient is less serious and clear-cut, the decision to speak up is more difficult.

Students should also take into account the probable effectiveness of speaking up. They are not obligated to speak up when they know that doing so will accomplish nothing. Yet they need to guard against rationalizing a policy of keeping quiet by supposing that speaking up will always be ineffective. It is difficult to know in advance whether voicing a concern will be effective. I personally know of cases where speaking up has made a difference, in matters ranging from the use of derogatory language to the proposed courses of surgery. Doubts about the effectiveness of speaking up should occasion not a retreat into silence but a search for the most effective way of voicing one's concerns.

When deciding whether to speak up, students may legitimately take into account the likely cost to themselves. They are not required to sacrifice their careers for some trivial matter, but neither should they keep quiet about a significant matter simply because speaking up may have some effect on their grades and careers. Obligations, by their very nature, require people to act in ways that sometimes include a cost or inconvenience to themselves.

Many students are concerned that speaking up will result in a lower grade than they deserve and that a lower grade will diminish their chances of getting into the residency program of their choice. Since the selection and self-selection of medical students tends to result in people who are exceedingly grade-conscious, it would not be surprising if many students exaggerated the role and importance of grades. There may, however, be times when speaking up will have some effect on students' grades. When an adverse effect is a real possibility, students may simply have to choose between doing what will maximize their grades and doing what fulfills their obligations in the broadest sense. In making this choice, students should try to examine their notion of a "good" residency. If a good residency is just a prestigious one, then students should recognize the importance they are assigning to prestige. But if a good residency is one that trains people to be good physicians, then students should recognize that there is something a little odd about choosing not to act as a good physician now in order to maximize their chances of later getting into a program that will train them to be good physicians.

The question of when students should speak up cannot be completely separated from the question of how students should speak up. In an obvious way the question of whether and when to speak up depends on what one is proposing to say and how one is going to say it. For example, students need very little cause or justification for asking about the medical indications of a particular procedure, whereas they need more cause or justification for going over a person's head.

When students have decided to speak directly to the person involved, there is still the question of how they should formulate their concerns. The phrasing and tone of what they say is more than a matter of style. Insofar as different ways of speaking up express different sensitivities, these ways are of ethical significance. Perhaps an example can illustrate this point.

Sometimes medical students notice a problem or make a diagnosis before the resident does. Students must then decide how, and how forcefully, to convey their discovery to the resident. They can even decide to play dumb: to tell the resident about some findings and tests so as to lead the resident to make the diagnosis that they have already made. Playing dumb may itself express various concerns or attitudes. Students may play dumb in order not to appear arrogant, to maintain a working relationship within a hierarchical system, or to get an egotistical person to see and act on the problem. Whether playing dumb expresses a kind of servility is an issue worth considering. Although patient care should be the primary concern, issues of attitude and character are not insignificant.

Learning how best to speak up is important because many of the problems that students encounter need to be resolved by talking to people face to face. Relatively few problems can or should be dealt with in other ways: by anonymous letters, note boxes, or grievance committees. The need for face-to-face engagement is not an unfortunate fact, but an occasion for developing a certain kind of character and work environment. It is an occasion for caring students to try to voice important concerns and disagreements in a way that does not alienate the people they are working with. This is a task that requires a lot of practice. Now is the time to begin.

### More Socratic

There are many reasons why students find it difficult to speak up. Some do not think it is their place or job to do so. Some are concerned about possible adverse effects on their grades, particularly when doing clerkships in specialties they hope to enter. Some fear that they will be subjected to ridicule for asking a question or expressing a concern. Some learn that it is considered improper to criticize fellow physicians. Some want to be viewed as loyal to the team, and few want to be seen as a rat or tattletale.

In spite of the reasons that make it difficult for students to speak up, I have argued that they have an obligation to do so. But by focusing on students' obligations I did not mean to excuse the people above them. Speaking up is a problem for everyone in medicine, and those with more power and authority have a greater obligation to confront the problem. They have a responsibility to speak up and a responsibility to try to change the conditions that make it so difficult for those below them to speak up.

It will not be easy to transform fearful silence into concerned conversation, but that is what needs to be done. There is a need for people to question or report the obviously bad. And in cases that are less obvious, there is a need for people to initiate discussions about what is good. For example, in one of the cases depicted at the beginning of this paper, the student and the resident had doubts about the aggressive course of treatment being given a child dying of AIDS. Perhaps the attending physician's plan of treatment was well-founded and involved the parents in a meaningful way. Perhaps not. Perhaps he was just responding to discrete technical problems. When students (and residents) fail to express their concerns in a case like this, everyone stands to lose. The patient is subjected to a course of treatment that may not be good in a broad sense. The family may suffer more. The attending physician may never examine certain assumptions. Future patients may face similar problems. And the students will fail to exercise and develop important habits of a caring physician.

I guess I am really suggesting that the practice of medicine needs to become more Socratic. Perhaps medicine could not function if everyone acted like Socrates—perhaps there would be too much discussion and too little patient care. Yet I believe that medicine could function quite well if everyone were a little more Socratic, a little more willing to raise questions about what is right and good.

## Notes

I would like to thank William Ruddick and Arthur Zitrin for their comments and encouragement. I would also like to thank the many medical students who have contributed to my education.

1   This account was suggested by Anna Barrett.
2   This account was suggested by Stacey Lane.
3   This account was suggested by Michelle Barry.
4   This account was suggested by Susan Staugaitis.
5   This account was suggested by Bartley Bryt.
6   Melvin Konner, *Becoming a Doctor* (New York: Penguin Books, 1987).
7   E. Haavi Morreim, "Am I My Brother's Warden? Responding to the Unethical or Incompetent Colleague," *Hastings Center Report* 23, no. 3 (1993): 19–27.
8   See, for example, John Rawls, *A Theory of Justice* (Cambridge, Mass.: Harvard University Press, 1971), 113–115.
9   A number of philosophers have written about the nature and importance of habit. Three prominent examples are Aristotle, John Dewey, and Maurice Merleau-Ponty. Aristotle discusses habituation in Book 2 of *Nichomachean Ethics*. Dewey devotes one part of *Human Nature and Conduct* (New York: Modern Library, 1957) to a consideration of habit. Merleau-Ponty discusses habit and the habitual body in *Phenomenology of Perception*. My own remarks on habit follow Dewey.
10  In a different context, Carol Gilligan says that the problem "becomes one of limiting responsibilities without abandoning moral concern." See *In a Different Voice* (Cambridge, Mass.: Harvard University Press, 1982), 21.

## Perspective Shift
Daniel Shapiro

He looks so sad, so forlorn. He chews a lip as he studies his sneakers. His hands clasp together and then awkwardly separate like uncomfortable acquaintances. His foot drums to a beat internal and irregular. His forehead sweats. The pen in his hand has been chewed and gnawed. Little tooth rivulets carpet its plastic veneer.

I have seen this clinical presentation a thousand times.

The helplessness has surfaced. He can no longer suppress it. He is a steam whistle, and the anxiety at facing cancer's horrible ambiguity has finally rumbled to the surface, erupting with volcanic emotional chaos. He expected better news.

We are staring at chest films that tell a sobering story. A tumor sits in the middle of the chest. An eight-centimeter mass. East to west it is smaller than it was the last time a scan was taken. North to south it appears longer. We both know that nodular sclerosing Hodgkin tumors can leave behind scar tissue. No one can tell if the tumor on this film is alive with cancerous intent or if what we see is a ghostly image of a beast now dead. The oracle of science, on this dry, cold winter day, is silent.

He paces slowly around the large windowed office, lost in thought, unable to find the words to describe his frustration with the unknown. It is painful to watch. These monthly scans have been challenging for him—they've provided so little evidence of progress to encourage the continued fight. Where will the energy come from for more aggressive chemotherapy? More nausea and fatigue? More restless nights?

He is young. He has had little experience with events not in his control.

Daniel Shapiro, "Perspective Shift," from *Journal of the American Medical Association*, vol. 279, 500. © 1998 by the American Medical Association. Reprinted by permission of the publisher.

He was brought up on simple just-world ethics. Phrases like "What goes around comes around" pepper his speech, and he is always telling me to go see the latest movie portraying a hero surmounting all odds. In his world, good people pull themselves out of poverty and despair and bad ones inevitably pay back in blood for every ridiculing utterance, every nip of ego they've displayed. He cannot reconcile his goodness with today's misfortunes.

I remain silent. He needs to learn to live with the ambiguity. To live, despite the ambiguity. He must come to these understandings on his own. I cannot show him the way. Nor will I offer false hope to make us feel better in this fleeting moment.

Of course I'll be here for him. It's the least I can do. After all, I need him. He is my young doctor and that is my tumor taunting us from the scan.

## Facing Our Mistakes
David Hilfiker

Looking at the appointment book for July 12, 1978, I notice that Barb Daily will be in today for her first prenatal examination. "Wonderful," I think, remembering my joy as I helped her deliver her first child two years ago. Barb and her husband Russ are friends, and our relationship became much closer with the shared experience of that birth. With so much exposure to disease every day in my rural family practice, I look forward to today's appointment with Barb and to the continuing relationship over the next months.

Barb seems to be in good health with all the symptoms and signs of pregnancy, but her urine pregnancy test is negative. I reassure Barb and myself that she is fine and that the test just hasn't turned positive yet. Rescheduling another test for the following week, I congratulate her on her condition and promise to get all her test results to her promptly.

But the next urine test is negative, too, which leaves me troubled. Isn't Barb pregnant? Has she had a missed abortion? I could make sure right now, of course, by ordering an ultrasound, but the new examination is available only in Duluth, 110 miles away from our northern Minnesota village, and it is expensive. I am aware of the Dailys' modest income. Besides, by waiting a few weeks, I'll find out for sure without the ultrasound. I call Barb on the phone and tell her about the negative test, about the possible abortion, and about the necessity of a repeat appointment in a few weeks if her next menstrual period does not occur on schedule.

It is, as usual, a hectic summer, and I almost forget about Barb's situation until a month later when she returns. Still no menstrual period, no abortion. She is confused and upset, since, she says, "I feel so pregnant." I

David Hilfiker, "Facing Our Mistakes," from *New England Journal of Medicine*, vol. 310, 118–122. © 1984 by the Massachusetts Medical Society. Reprinted by permission of the publisher.

am bothered, too, especially because her uterus continues to be enlarged. Her urine test remains definitely negative.

I break the bad news to her. "I think you have a missed abortion. You were probably pregnant, but the baby appears to have died some weeks ago, before your first examination. Unfortunately, you didn't have the miscarriage to get rid of the dead tissue from the baby and the placenta. If a miscarriage does not occur within a few weeks, I'd recommend a re-examination, another pregnancy test, and if nothing shows up, a dilation and curettage to clean out the uterus."

Barb is disappointed and saddened; there are tears. Both she and Russ have sufficient background in science to understand the technical aspects of the situation, but that doesn't alleviate the sorrow. We talk in the office at some length and make an appointment for two weeks later.

When Barb returns, Russ is with her. Still no menstrual period, no miscarriage, and a negative pregnancy test. It is difficult, but it also feels right to be able to share in friends' sadness. Thoroughly reviewing the situation with both of them, I schedule the D and C for later in the week.

Friday morning, when Barb is wheeled into the operating room, we chat before she is put to sleep. The surgical nurses in our small hospital are all friends, too, so the atmosphere is warm and relaxed. After induction of anesthesia, I examine Barb's pelvis. To my hands, the uterus now seems bigger than it had two days previously, but since all the pregnancy tests were negative, the uterus couldn't have grown. I continue the operation.

But this morning there is considerably more blood than usual, and it is only with great difficulty that I am able to extract any tissue. The body parts I remove are much larger than I had expected, considering when the fetus died, and they are not the decomposing tissue I'd anticipated. These are body parts that were recently alive! I suppress the rising panic in my body and try to complete the procedure. I am unable to evacuate the uterus completely, however, and after much sweat and worry, I stop, hoping that the uterus will expel the rest within a few days.

Russ is waiting outside the operating room, so I sit with him for a few minutes, telling him that Barb is fine but that there were some problems with the procedure. Since I haven't completely thought through what has happened, I can't be very helpful in answering his questions. I leave hurriedly for the office, promising to return that afternoon to talk with them once Barb has recovered from the anesthesia.

In between seeing other patients in the office that morning, I make several rushed phone calls, trying to figure out what has happened. Despite reassurances from the pathologist that it is statistically "impossible" for four consecutive pregnancy tests to be negative during a viable pregnancy, the horrifying awareness is growing that I have probably aborted Barb's living child. I won't know for sure until several days later, when the pathology report is available. In a daze I walk over to the hospital and try to tell Russ and Barb as much as I know, without telling them all that I suspect. I tell them that there may be more tissue expelled and that I won't know for sure about the pregnancy until the next week.

I can't really face my own suspicions yet.

That weekend I receive a tearful call from Barb. She has just passed some recognizable body parts of the baby; what is she to do? The bleeding has stopped, and she feels physically well, so it is apparent that the abortion I began on Friday is now over. I schedule a time in midweek to meet with them and review the entire situation.

The pathology report confirms my worst fears: I have aborted a living fetus at about 13 weeks of age. No explanation can be found for the negative pregnancy tests. My consultation with Barb and Russ later in the week is one of the hardest things I have ever done. Fortunately, their scientific sophistication allows me to describe in some detail what I have done and what my rationale was. But nothing can obscure the hard reality: I have killed their baby.

Politely, almost meekly, Russ asks whether the ultrasound examination could not have helped us. It almost seems that he is trying to protect my feelings, trying to absolve me of some of the responsibility. "Yes," I answer, "if I had ordered the ultrasound, we would have known that the baby was alive." I cannot explain to him why I didn't recommend it.

Over the next days and weeks and months, my guilt and anger grow. I discuss the events with my partners, with our pathologist, and with obstetric specialists. Some of my mistakes are obvious: I relied too heavily on one particular test; I was not skillful in determining the size of the uterus by pelvic examination; I should have ordered the ultrasound before proceeding with the D and C. Other mistakes become apparent as we review my handling of the case. There is simply no way I can justify what I have done. To make matters worse, complications after the D and C have caused much discomfort, worry, and expense. Barb is unable to become pregnant again for two years.

As physicians our automatic response to reading about such a tragedy is to try to discover what went wrong, to analyze why the mistakes occurred, and to institute corrective measures so that such things do not happen again. This response is important, indeed necessary, and I spent hours in such a review. But it is inadequate if it does not address our own emotional and spiritual experience of the events.

Although I was as honest with the Dailys as I could be in those next months, although I told them everything they wanted to know and described to them as completely as I could what had happened, I never shared with them the agony that I underwent trying to deal with the reality of the events. I never did ask for their forgiveness. I felt somehow that they had enough sorrow without having to bear my burden as well. Somehow, I felt, it was my responsibility to deal with my guilt alone.

Everyone, of course, makes mistakes, and no one enjoys the consequences. But the potential consequences of our medical mistakes are so overwhelming that it is almost impossible for practicing physicians to deal with their errors in a psychologically healthy fashion. Most people—doctors and patients alike—harbor deep within themselves the expectation that the physician will be perfect. No one seems prepared to accept the simple fact of life that physicians, like anyone else, will make mistakes.

By the very nature of our work, we physicians daily make decisions of extreme gravity. Our work in the intensive-care unit, in the emergency room, in the surgery suite, or in the delivery room offers us hundreds of opportunities daily to miscalculate, often with drastic consequences.

And it is not only in these settings but also in the humdrum of routine daily care that a physician can blunder into tragedy. One evening, for instance, a local boy was brought to the emergency room after an apparently minor automobile accident. One leg and foot were injured, but he was otherwise fine. After examining him, I consulted by telephone with an orthopedic surgeon in Duluth, and we decided that I would try to correct what appeared on the X-ray film to be a dislocated foot. As usual, I offered the patient and his mother (who happened to be a nurse with whom I worked regularly) a choice: I could reduce the dislocation in our small hospital or they could travel to Duluth to see the specialist. I was somewhat offended when they decided they would go to Duluth. My feelings changed considerably when the surgeon called me the next morning to thank me for the referral. He reported that the patient had not had a dislocation at all but a severe posterior compartment syndrome, which had hyperflexed the foot, causing it to appear dislocated. The posterior compartment had required immediate surgery the previous night in order to save the muscles of the lower leg. I felt physically weak as I realized that this young man would have been permanently injured had his mother not decided on her own to take him to Duluth.

Although much less drastic than the threat of death or severe disability, perhaps the most frequent result of physician misjudgment is the wasting of money, often in large amounts. Every practicing physician spends thousands of dollars of patients' money every day in the costs for visits, laboratory examinations, medications, and hospitalizations. An unneeded examination, the needless admission of a patient to the hospital, even the unnecessary advice to stay home from work can waste large amounts of money—frequently, the money of people who have little to spare. One comes to feel that any decision may have important consequences.

The cumulative impact of such mistakes (and the ever-present potential for many others) has had a devastating effect on my own emotional health, as it does, I believe, for most physicians. For it is not only the obvious mistakes with obvious results that trouble us. Such mistakes as I made with Barb are fortunately rare occurrences for any physician, and an emotionally mature person may learn to cope with them. But there are also those frequent times when an obvious mistake may lead to less obvious consequences, when the physician errs in judgment, never to know how important the error was.

Some years ago, as I was rushing to an imminent delivery, a young woman stopped me in the hospital hall to tell me that her mother had been having chest pains all night. Should she be brought to the emergency room? I knew her mother well, had examined her the previous week, and knew of her recurring angina. "No," I responded, thinking primarily of my busy schedule and the fact that I was already an hour late because of the unexpected delivery. "Take her over to the office, and I'll see her there as soon as I'm done here." It would be a lot more convenient to see her in the office, I thought. About 20 minutes later, as I was finishing the delivery, our clinic nurse rushed into the delivery room, her face pale and frantic. "Come quick! Mrs. Martin just collapsed." I sprinted the 100 yards to the office to find Mrs. Martin in cardiac arrest. Like many physician offices at that time, ours was not equipped with the advanced life-support equipment necessary to handle the situation. Despite everything we could do, Mrs. Martin died.

Would she have survived if I had initially agreed to see her in the emergency room where the requisite staff and equipment were available? No one will ever know for sure, but I have to live with the possibility that she might have lived if I had made a routine decision differently, a decision similar to many others I would make that day, yet one with such an overwhelming outcome.

There is also the common situation of the seriously ill, hospitalized patient who requires almost continuous decision making on the part of the physician. Although no "mistake" may be evident, there are always things that could have been done better: a little more of this medication, starting that treatment a little earlier, recognizing this complication a bit sooner, limiting the number of visitors, and so forth. If the patient dies, the physician is left wondering whether the care provided was adequate. There is no way to be certain, for no one can know what would have happened if things had been done differently. Usually, in fact, it is difficult to get an honest opinion from consultants and other physicians about what one could have done differently. (Judge not, that you not be judged?) In the end, the physician has to swallow the concern, suppress the guilt, and move on to the next patient. He or she may simply be unable to discover whether the mistakes were responsible for the patient's death.

Worst of all, the possibility of a serious mistake is present with each patient the physician sees. The inherent uncertainty of medical practice creates a situation in which errors are always possible. Was that baby I just sent home with a diagnosis of a mild viral fever actually in the early stages of a serious meningitis? Could that nine-year-old with stomach cramps whose mother I just lectured about psychosomatic illness come into the hospital tomorrow with a ruptured appendix? Indeed, the closest I have ever come to involvement in a courtroom malpractice case was the result of my treatment of an apparently minor wrist injury one week after it happened: I misread a straightforward X-ray film and sent the young boy home with a diagnosis of sprain. I next heard about it five years later, when after being summoned to a hearing, I discovered that the fracture I had missed had not healed, and the patient had required extensive treatment and difficult surgery years later.

As practicing primary-care physicians, then, we work in an impossible situation. Each of the myriad decisions to be made every day has the potential for drastic consequences if it is not determined properly. And it is highly likely that sooner or later we will make the mistake that kills or seriously injures another person. How can we live with that knowledge? And after a serious mistake has been made, how can we continue in daily practice and expose ourselves again? How can we who see ourselves as healers deal with such guilt?

Painfully, almost unbelievably, we physicians are even less prepared to deal with our mistakes than the average lay person is. The climate of medical school and residency training, for instance, makes it nearly impossible to confront the emotional consequences of mistakes; it is an environment in which precision seems to predominate. In the large centers where doctors are trained, teams of physicians discuss the smallest details of cases; teaching is usually conducted to make it seem "obvious" what decisions should have been made. And when a physician does make an important mistake, it is first whispered about in the halls, as if it were a sin. Much later, a case conference is called in which experts who have had weeks to think about the situation discuss the way it should have been handled. The environment in which physicians are trained does not encourage them to talk about their mistakes or about their emotional responses to them.

Indeed, errors are rarely admitted or discussed once a physician is in private practice. I have some indication from consultants and colleagues that I am of at least average competence as a physician. The mistakes I have discussed here represent only a fraction of those of which I am aware. I assume that my colleagues at my own clinic and elsewhere are responsible for similar numbers of major and minor errors. Yet we rarely discuss them; I cannot remember a single instance in which another physician initiated a discussion of a mistake for the purpose of clarifying his or her own emotional response or deciding how to follow up. (I do not wish to imply that we don't discuss difficult cases or unfortunate results; yet these discussions are always handled so delicately in the presence of the "offending" physician that there is simply no space for confession or absolution.)

The medical profession simply seems to have no place for its mistakes. There is no permission given to talk about errors, no way of venting emotional responses. Indeed, one would almost think that mistakes are in the same category as sins: it is permissible to talk about them only when they happen to other people.

If the profession has no room for its mistakes, society seems to have even more rigid expectations of its physicians. The malpractice situation in our country is symptomatic of this attitude. In what other profession are practitioners regularly sued for hundreds of thousands of dollars because of a misjudgment? A lawyer informed me I could be sued for $50,000 for misreading the X-ray film that led to the young man's unhealed fracture. I am sure the Dailys could have successfully sued me for large amounts of money, had they chosen to do so. Experienced physicians who are honest with themselves can count many potential malpractice suits against them. Even the word "malpractice" carries the implication that one has done something more than make a natural mistake; it connotes guilt and sinfulness.

It is easy, of course, to understand why this situation has arisen. These mistakes are terrible; their consequences are drastic; and the victim or family should be compensated for medical bills, time lost from work, and suffering or death. But in our society, rather than establish a "patient compensation fund" (similar to worker's compensation) from which a deserving patient can be compensated for an injury that results from a legitimate mistake, we insist that the doctor be sued for "malpractice," judged guilty, and forced to compensate the patient personally. An atmosphere of denial is created: the "good physician" doesn't make mistakes.

The drastic consequences of our mistakes, the repeated opportunities to make them, the uncertainty about our own culpability when results are poor, and the medical and societal denial that mistakes must happen all result in an intolerable paradox for the physician. We see the horror of our own mistakes, yet we are given no permission to deal with their enormous emotional impact; instead, we are forced to continue the routine of repeatedly making decisions, any one of which could lead us back into the same pit.

Perhaps the only adequate avenue for dealing with this paradox is spiritual. Although mistakes are not usually sins, they engender similar feelings of guilt. How can I not feel guilty about the death of Barb's baby, the lack of adequate emergency care for Mrs. Martin, the fracture that didn't heal? Whether I "ought" to feel guilty is a moot point; most of us do feel guilty under such circumstances.

The only real answer for guilt is spiritual confession, restitution, and absolution. Yet within the structure of modern medicine there is simply no place for this spiritual healing. Although the emotionally mature physician may find it possible to give the patient or family a clinical description of what happened, the technical details are often so difficult for the lay person to understand that the nature of the mistake is hidden. Or if an error is clearly described, it is presented as "natural," "understandable," or "unavoidable" (which, indeed, it often is). But there is no place for real confession: "This is the mistake I made; I'm sorry." How can one say that to a grieving mother, to a family that has lost a member? It simply doesn't fit into the physician-patient relationship.

Even if one were bold enough to consider such a confession, strong voices would raise objections. When I finally heard about the unhealed fracture in my young patient, I was anxious that the incident not create antagonism between me and the family, since we live in a small town and see each other frequently. I was tempted to call the family and express my apologies and the hope that a satisfactory settlement could be worked out. I mentioned that possibility to a malpractice lawyer, but he was strongly opposed, urging me not to have any contact with the family until a settlement was reached. Even if a malpractice suit is not likely, the nature of the physician-patient relationship makes such a reversal of roles "unseemly." Can I further burden an already grieving family with the complexities of my feelings, my burden?

And if confession is difficult, what are we to say about restitution? The very nature of our work means that we are dealing with elements that cannot be restored in any meaningful way. What can I offer the Dailys in restitution?

I have not been successful in dealing with the paradox. Any patient encounter can dump me back into the situation of having caused more harm than good, yet my role is to be a healer. Since there has been no permission to address the paradox openly, I lapse into neurotic behavior to deal with my anxiety and guilt. Little wonder that physicians are accused of having a God complex; little wonder that we are defensive about our judgments; little wonder that we blame the patient or the previous physician when things go wrong, that we yell at the nurses for their mistakes, that we have such high rates of alcoholism, drug addiction, and suicide.

At some point we must bring our mistakes out of the closet. We need to give ourselves permission to recognize our errors and their consequences. We need to find healthy ways to deal with our emotional responses to those errors. Our profession is difficult enough without our having to wear the yoke of perfection.

## God at the Bedside

Jerome Groopman

Not long ago, in the oncology clinic where I work, my patient Anna Angelo asked me to pray to God. At the time, prayer was far from the forefront of my mind. Anna (her name has been changed to maintain confidentiality) is a 71-year-old woman from Boston's North End with long-standing cardiac and hepatobiliary disease. Six years ago, breast cancer developed. The tumor was incurable from the time of diagnosis, since it had already spread to bone. The cancer cells tested positive for estrogen and progesterone receptors, and Anna was treated with a series of hormonal agents, which, over the ensuing years, largely controlled the disease. A devout Catholic, she regularly attended Mass and counted her priest among her closest friends. "God has been good to me," Anna said at the end of each visit.

Over the previous two months, Anna had been complaining to her internist about loss of appetite and fatigue. He ordered blood tests and then a CAT scan. The cancer had metastasized to her liver. A biopsy showed that the hepatic metastases no longer expressed hormone receptors. When Anna arrived for her appointment with me, she had already been informed of her biopsy results. The first thing she said was that she wanted to live as long as possible but was concerned about the toll of chemotherapy.

I explained that the choice of a treatment plan would not be simple, given her complicating medical problems. Many of the drugs could have serious side effects on her heart and would be metabolized by her liver. So, before recommending a regimen, I would consult with her internist, car-

Jerome Groopman, "God at the Bedside," from *New England Journal of Medicine*, vol. 350, 1176–1178. © 2004 by the Massachusetts Medical Society. Reprinted by permission of the publisher.

diologist, and gastroenterologist. Anna took in my words and then said, "Doctor, I'm frightened. I pray every day. I want you to pray for me."

Anna looked squarely at me. It was clear she wanted a response. For a long while, I did not know what to say. A doctor's words have great power for a patient; they can help to heal, and they can do great harm. The specialty of oncology routinely involves treating people who are in dire circumstances and find themselves facing their own mortality. Many of my patients seek strength and solace in their faith.

None of the training I received in medical school, residency, fellowship, or practice had taught me how to reply to Anna. And although I am religious, I consider my beliefs and prayers a private matter. Should I sidestep Anna's request, in effect distancing myself from her at a moment of great need? Or should I cross the boundary from the purely professional to the personal and join her in prayer?

Dilemmas like this one have become points of sharp contention in the medical world. How should doctors examine and engage religion in the lives of their patients and in their own lives as clinicians? Is there any place for God at the bedside during rounds?

The United States is a deeply religious country, and several surveys show both that a large majority of patients want physicians to be engaged in their spiritual lives and that the sick believe in miraculous healing when medicine can offer no proven cure. But religious beliefs are not always positive or beneficial. One of my most instructive experiences of the effects of religious belief occurred some three decades ago, when I was a third-year medical student. An Orthodox Jewish woman in her 20s was admitted to the surgical service with a large breast mass. She seemed intelligent and animated, and it made no sense to me that she would have ignored a growth in her breast that was the size of a walnut. In my naïveté, I thought that our shared heritage positioned me to communicate with her in a particularly effective way, and I encouraged her to confide in me the reason why she had let the mass grow so large before seeking a surgeon. It turned out that she had had an affair with her employer, and she saw her tumor as God's punishment for her sin. There was no hope for her, no reason to continue living, because her death was God's will.

I was in over my head. I had brashly treaded into theological territory without a clinical compass. Was her confession meant as a call for absolution or a confirmation of her transgression? It was not my place to afford either, and with a mix of confusion and shame, I retreated from her. Later, she shared her secret with the attending surgeon. I never knew what he had said to her that convinced her to be treated. Nor, during my subsequent medical training, was I ever taught how to speak to patients about matters of faith.

Centuries ago, when healers came primarily from the ranks of monks, rabbis, and imams, and when nurses were nuns or members of religious orders, there was no clear divide between biology and acts of God in the genesis of an illness or between the physical and spiritual components of its treatment. In the modern era, religion and science are understood to be sharply divided, the two occupying very different domains. Religion explores the nature of God and offers rituals for implementing God's will, whereas science eschews any such metaphysics and through experimentation unveils the workings of the material world.

But in the minds of many of our patients, there is no such schism. Religion, perhaps more than any other single force, can sculpt the experience of illness. In America today, religious influence can go beyond concepts embodied in the three Abrahamic faiths. Some patients and their doctors have turned to Eastern philosophies, seeking to integrate Buddhist, Taoist, and Ayurvedic ideas and practices into clinical care.

Different faiths dictate different forms of behavior, social interactions, and views about how to live and how to die. For this reason, some medical educators have argued that religion is a clinical variable to be considered in every case and that a "spiritual history" should become a regular part of the patient interview. Indeed, such a history may yield key diagnostic clues or guide recommendations about disease prevention and suggest strategies to ensure compliance with treatment. But if this kind of history taking becomes common practice, when, by whom, and how should it be done? At the first visit, or only after a close bond has been formed between patient and doctor? By the medical student, resident, or attending physician? And how would doctors manage the theological fallout?

Many doctors, understandably, are leery of moving outside the strictly clinical and venturing into the spiritual realm. As was clear in the case of the Orthodox woman I met as a student, theologies can sometimes be toxic. Religion can be a wellspring of great strength and comfort or a pool of guilt and pain. If we begin taking a spiritual history, then we risk becoming clinical judges of what we hear. But although doctors should not presume to take on the mantle of the clergy, I believe that they cannot always avoid evaluating whether the personal religious beliefs of their patients are salubrious. Unfortunately, this type of evaluation requires deeper knowledge of different religions and their clinically beneficial and harmful conceptions than most of us possess. Venturing into the spiritual domain also means confronting a patient's expectations about the outcome of an illness, particularly what it means not to be cured despite faith and prayer. If a patient prays for a medical miracle and it doesn't occur, does that mean that God doesn't love her or that she is unworthy because her will and character were too weak to exert the "power of prayer"? Popular culture makes much of the ability of will and faith to miraculously overcome dreaded diseases for which modern medicine has no proven remedies. Rigorous documentation of such widely touted spontaneous remissions is scant, and even in those rare true cases, cause and effect are obscure.

A doctor's practice can also be influenced, consciously or subconsciously, by his own religious beliefs. Moreover, his own faith, like that of his patients, may be tested by the trauma and travail that he witnesses. I came from a home where faith was strong but not fundamentalist, where belief coexisted with doubt. After spending six weeks on a pediatric oncology ward at a time when most children with cancer died terrible deaths, I was on the verge of losing my faith. Theodicy, the question of why a benevolent God would permit such suffering in the universe, can be brought into sharp focus in the hospital. The intimacy of the physician-patient dialogue could cause this question to emerge. What if Anna had asked me why God had chosen her to suffer? Should a doctor participate in such a dialogue?

Even as we ponder whether or how we should step inside the religious worlds of our patients, we should also ask whether members of the clergy should enter more deeply into our clinical sphere. There is a great imbalance of power between patient and doctor. Often, I have been insensitive to this imbalance and have taken a patient's silence to represent tacit assent to my recommendations. A member of the clergy can speak to a doctor at eye level and act as an advocate for a patient who may be intimidated by a physician and reluctant to question or oppose his or her advice. A priest, a rabbi, or an imam can help patients to determine which clinical options are in concert with their religious imperatives and can give the physician the language with which to address the patient's spiritual needs.

Facing Anna, I searched for a response. I reminded myself that whenever I wear that white coat I am a physician and that whatever I say or do should be for the clinical benefit of my patient. I briefly pondered the question of whether prayer was "good for health." This issue had captured the public's imagination, but published research on the subject was often preliminary and inconclusive. It was a legitimate and intriguing subject of scientific inquiry, but somehow, at the moment, it seemed remote from what Anna was asking for—a heartfelt answer.

And so, unsure of where to fix the boundary between the professional and the personal, unsure what words were appropriate, I drew on the Talmudic custom of my ancestors and the pedagogical practice of my mentors and answered her question with a question.

"What is the prayer you want?"

"Pray for God to give my doctors wisdom," Anna said.

To that, I silently echoed, "Amen."

# PART III

**Health Care Ethics
and the Clinician's Role**

## Glossary of Basic Ethical Concepts
## in Health Care and Research
Nancy M. P. King

*Autonomy.* The principle of respect for autonomy, and the right of self-determination, are important concepts in health care ethics. "Autonomy" means the ability to govern oneself and the freedom to do so. "Self-determination" is often used to mean autonomy, especially in health care settings.

A person acts autonomously if that person acts intentionally, with understanding, and without being controlled by others. Both persons and their actions can be autonomous; autonomous people do not always act autonomously, and sometimes people who are not autonomous are able to make autonomous decisions or act autonomously in some instances. It is important to remember that no one is "fully" autonomous; we judge autonomy by the expectations we have of common human behavior, and set a minimal standard of "substantial" autonomy by which to judge people and their actions.

In health care, respecting autonomy does not mean simply laying out all the options and telling the patient, "You decide." Respecting patients' autonomy often includes promoting an individual's ability to deliberate effectively, for example by providing a recommendation and discussing the reasons behind it.

Autonomy is not the same as freedom, and usually we view autonomy as including some responsibility for the consequences of one's actions. Now that society has become especially concerned about the interests or rights of communities, there is much disagreement about the boundaries between an individual's autonomy and the legitimate rights or interests of others.

Competence and decisional capacity, concepts related to autonomy, are defined below.

*Beneficence/Best Interests.* The principle of beneficence, or the best interests of the person, is often contrasted to autonomy. There may, for example, be times when a health care provider believes that what an autonomous patient wants is not in that person's best interests. Beneficence focuses on doing good. The crucial question is, who should be allowed to judge what is good? An individual, health care providers, family members, friends, and other authorities may all have different judgments about what is in the individual's best interests. Best interests may be defined narrowly, as in "best medical interests," or broadly enough to consider a wide variety of personal factors and values.

The Hippocratic maxim "Above all, do no harm" is technically an injunction to *nonmaleficence*—avoiding harm—rather than to beneficence—doing good. In health care, these principles are often closely related and considered together. If they are ranked in importance, nonmaleficence generally comes first; however, as you might imagine, health care providers and patients must often weigh the risk of doing harm against the chance of doing good when deciding about treatment.

How "harm" is defined and who defines it are problems for nonmaleficence, just as they are for beneficence. At least one significant difference exists between the two concepts: physicians and other health care providers sometimes assert the right not to cause harm by withdrawing from the care of a patient and substituting another caregiver. A parallel unilateral right to do good against the patient's will does not exist.

*Coercion.* Coercion is control of one person's behavior by another. It is always incompatible with autonomy and is therefore morally unacceptable, unless it can be justified by a principle or interest that is sufficiently compelling to outweigh autonomy under the circumstances—for example, the safety of other persons put at grave risk by an autonomous actor.

Actions may be coercive, but coercion is usually accomplished by threats. Many influences are loosely called coercive, but "coercion" should be reserved for influences that are intended to control behavior by means of a severe and irresistible threat. Coerced actions are intentional actions, but actions about which the actor "has no choice." Controversy can arise about coercion in two areas: Generally, how should we define and measure what is "irresistible"? And specifically, can *offers* be so irresistible as to be coercive? (For example, is the promise of parole for a prisoner who submits to medical experimentation so great an offer as to overwhelm the person's reasonable concerns about the safety of the experiment and inclination to say no?)

Sometimes people talk about coercive situations. Unpleasant circumstances can indeed make people feel that they have no choice, but only other people can be coercive, because only other people can intend to influence that person's behavior. For example, the situation of having a severe mental illness can make a person feel that s/he has no choice but to take a dangerous drug with unpleasant side effects. That person is not coerced by the situation. But if taking the drug is required as a qualification for receiving government assistance in housing or education, such requirements—since they are instituted with the intention of encouraging mentally ill people to stay on medication—may be (but are not necessarily) coercive.

Manipulation and persuasion must be distinguished from coercion. They are each defined below.

*Competence.* A legal term. Adults (people age 18 and over) are presumed competent until proven otherwise. Thus, a severely impaired adult who has not been legally determined to be incompetent is legally competent. The determination of incompetence is made in a legal proceeding and can be quite complex and detailed. A determination may be global or limited. Someone of limited competence may retain some legal decision-making rights while losing others. For example, a limited guardianship might be established for financial matters, but the person would retain the legal right to make health care decisions. Involuntary commitment is not the same as a determination of incompetence. "Competence" is often mistakenly considered synonymous with "decisional capacity," which is not a legal term. It is defined below.

*Confidentiality.* Confidentiality is the duty, expectation, and/or promise that information exchanged within a relationship will not be spread beyond the boundaries of that relationship (that is, "keeping secrets"). Confidentiality causes problems because so many different relationships can be connected to a confidential relationship. Sometimes a potential need arises to protect others who might need to know confidential information (for example, landlords or employers). Sometimes the perceived need may be to share confidential information with others (for example, family or health care providers) who could benefit the person who expects confidentiality to be maintained. Sorting out and balancing these competing needs and interests can be extremely difficult.

Confidentiality is not the same as privacy, which is defined below.

*Conflict of Interest.* A general term that calls attention to a variety of ethical problems in service relationships. People who find themselves caught in a conflict of interest may feel that they are trying unsuccessfully to serve two masters or that they have conflicting loyalties or duties to others. (For example, managed care has given rise to much concern about conflicts of interest, because physicians in managed care contracts have incentives to save money that may conflict with their duty of beneficence to patients. However, traditional "fee-for-service" medicine rewards physicians for delivering more services, which may conflict with the duty of nonmaleficence to patients.)

Often the first type of conflict we think of is financial, but there are many others. For example, a parent's decisions about one child may be affected by the needs of the other children in the family; a health care provider may be concerned about the competing needs of family members other than the patient, or about how to meet the needs of more than one patient when time is limited; and there are many others. The term "conflict of interest" helps us flag complicated situations and sort out the potentially competing needs and interests involved.

Conflicts of interest are common in life and at least some may be unavoidable. How they should be addressed depends on the circumstances. Sometimes they should be eliminated; other times, they may be "managed," for example, by an oversight mechanism; and sometimes, disclosing them may be sufficient to allow the persons potentially affected by them to respond appropriately to the risks they pose.

*Decisional Capacity.* The ability to make substantially autonomous decisions. It is assumed that adults have it. When questions arise about someone's decisional capacity, it is measured using practicality and common sense, and with reference to the specific decision(s) at issue. For example, an impaired person might have the capacity to decide about going into a nursing home but lack the ability to choose between two treatments for a health problem because that requires greater reasoning skills.

Although sometimes with mental illness, decisional capacity may need to be assessed by an expert, such as a psychiatrist, in most cases an equally reliable determination can be made by those who know the person, have talked with him or her, and are familiar with the circumstances. The best test of someone's capacity to make a particular decision is going through the informed consent process. A variety of different standards can then be used; they range from very lenient (does the person appear to express a choice?), to the overly strict (does the person make the "right" decision for the "right" reasons?). A more appropriate standard is provided by the definition of substantial autonomy given above: Does this person seem to know that there is a choice to be made, and does s/he seem to be choosing intentionally, with understanding of the meaning and consequences of the choice, and without being controlled by others? Difficult questions can arise about when the nonlegal determination that someone lacks decisional capacity should be followed up by a legal determination about competence.

*Justice.* Justice is a significant ethical principle that has many different aspects. Generally speaking, we worry about justice on a larger scale than the individual—for example, for communities, special groups (women, minorities, disabled persons, etc.), and societies. Justice is roughly synonymous with fairness, but what is just or fair depends on the circumstances. Is treating everyone equally just? Or is affirmative action more just because it redresses past wrongs? Distributive justice addresses how social goods (like food, shelter, and health care) should be distributed. Once again, we might ask whether equality is a just principle of distribution, or whether "from each according to his ability, to each according to his needs" is more just. Fair procedures and fair hearings are also components of justice.

*Manipulation.* Manipulation is the hardest category to grasp in the trio of coercion, manipulation, and persuasion. Manipulation falls in between the other two and can essentially be one of two things: an intentional and successful alteration of a person's available choices by means that are not coercive (for example, by a resistible threat or offer), or an intentional and successful alteration of a person's perception of those choices by means that are not persuasive, that is, not focused on reason (for example, by a successful appeal to emotion, or by psychological influence). A common health care example is when a provider mistakenly believes that persuasion is morally wrong, but believes that a particular choice is the right one for a patient, and therefore slants or selectively provides information, perhaps using language chosen for a particular emotional effect, in order to ensure that the informed consent process has the outcome desired by the provider. A common example outside of health care is advertising.

Manipulation is to a large extent a matter of degree and a question of context. It is not always incompatible with autonomy, but there are almost always alternatives that help to protect, promote, and foster autonomy, which manipulation definitely does not.

*Paternalism.* "Paternalism" is another term that is often loosely used. True paternalism, also called strong paternalism, occurs when one person overrides the autonomous choices and actions of another in the other person's best interests (for example, preventing a "rational suicide"). It is not paternalistic to override someone's actions or choices in order to benefit, or prevent harm to, third parties. It is also not paternalistic to override someone's actions or choices when that person is not acting autonomously (for example, preventing suicide by a person who is delusional), because then beneficence and autonomy are not in conflict. However, this is also often called paternalism, or weak paternalism. As the suicide examples given help to show, many occasions when "paternalism" is mentioned are instances where the autonomy and beneficence of the choices at issue are questionable or in dispute.

*Persuasion.* Persuasion is the intentional and successful attempt to induce a person, through appeals to reason, to freely adopt the beliefs, values, attitudes, intentions, or actions advocated by the persuader. It is compatible with autonomy, and indeed often facilitates autonomous decision making, because it is based on reasoned discourse and shared communication and discussion. Education and persuasion are closely linked.

*Privacy.* Privacy has two meanings: a common-sense meaning and a legal meaning. The constitutional right of privacy can be confusing because it means freedom from governmental intrusion into certain decisions and actions relating to one's body, relationships, reproduction, speech, and ideas—a real grab bag of personal actions and decisions. (This meaning of privacy has been somewhat modified by the courts, from a "constitutional privacy right" to a "constitutional liberty interest.")

Common-sense privacy is a somewhat different grab bag. It refers to freedom from intrusions upon solitude (being eavesdropped upon, photographed, or spied on in circumstances where we commonly have an "expectation of privacy," such as at home) and freedom from having private facts made public or from unwanted publicity (again, this is measured against what society reasonably believes is private and what is public). The privacy of medical records (more properly, the confidentiality of their contents, but popular and legislative language have confused the two) is an issue of growing importance in this information age, and determinations about what may and may not be shared with others (such as employers, insurers, and information purchasers) depends on what is considered a reasonable expectation of privacy.

"Privacy" in any of its meanings is not the same as "confidentiality," which means keeping shared information within a relationship.

*Rights.* The concept of rights in health care is overused and difficult to define, but needs clarification. Beginning in the 1960s and 1970s, American society became accustomed to talking about the rights of comparatively disadvantaged groups, such as ethnic and racial minorities, women, and patients. More recently, physicians and other health care professionals have pointed out that they have rights too (paralleling the development of "victims' rights" to complement the rights of persons accused and convicted of crimes). As the uses of the term "rights" have become more extensive, its meaning has faded. There are many different types of legal rights, for example, so that the mere assertion of a right tells us little about its scope or effect. Much specificity is necessary in order to make a claim of right clear and meaningful.

The best way to think about rights (moral or legal) is that they are correlative to duties. Thus, if I have a right to do X, someone else—an individual or perhaps the state—has a duty to me, either not to interfere with my doing X or, in some instances, to assist me in doing X. I may also have a duty to exercise my right responsibly, so as not to interfere with the rights of others.

One common problem with rights language is the perception that everyone has rights and no one has responsibilities. Another is that rights belong only to individuals, so that the rights of individuals are pitted against the interests of communities. Rights language should be used judiciously to avoid these pitfalls.

*Virtues.* Many of the basic concepts of ethics take the form of *principles*, that is, rules of general application. Autonomy, beneficence, and justice are all examples of principles. Rights also play a prominent role in medical ethics, because of the connections between ethics, policy, and law.

But there are other ways of conceptualizing ethics. One way that is well known to most of us is through virtues.

Virtue language is the language of "being" rather than "doing." Whereas principles provide "rules" for "solving" ethical "problems," virtues describe the kind of people we aspire to be. They set standards of character and consider how different traits of character add up to a good person, or a good health professional. The moral language that many people use more closely matches virtues than it does principles. A principlist might say, "You're wrong," or, "It's the right thing to do." Instead, many people say things like "I wouldn't feel right if I did that" or "I'm not the kind of person who could do that." Many codes of ethics for health care professionals use virtue language, focusing on what it means to be a good doctor or a good nurse more than on rules and action guides (for example, "The nurse should be honest" rather than "The nurse should tell the truth").

Virtue language is the language of many religious traditions and forms the basis of much of the moral instruction that families pass on to children, but the concept of virtue ethics also has roots in Aristotle. Any complete system of ethics will include both principles and virtues, seeing them as complementary rather than competing ways of conceptualizing ethics.

# Ethics in Medicine: An Introduction to Moral Tools and Traditions
Larry R. Churchill, Nancy M. P. King, and David Schenck

## Foreground Decisions in a Background of Relationships

In this volume the reader is confronted with a variety of complex ethical situations in medicine and health care. These situations are typically expressed as problems requiring sharp-edged, either/or moral choices: Should a physician lie to a patient when the lie promises patient benefit? Is it good to be candid about medical mistakes, and if so, whose good is served? Should physicians ever assist their terminally ill patients in suicide? Should patients' social status affect whether they receive a scarce, life-saving treatment, such as a heart transplant?

This essay is a brief introduction to ethics in medicine. One of its aims is to provide a sketch of the major ethical theories and moral traditions that are commonly used as tools for analyzing and resolving moral dilemmas. Although moral problem-solving is an important part of ethics, it is only a part. Apparently stark moral dilemmas often seem highlighted in ethics, but all such dilemmas stand before a background of understandings, relationships, and experiences that prefigure and shape them. Before and after such choices, ethics is about the nature and quality of human encounters. In this essay we will attend to both foreground and background considerations.

A physician who decides to lie to her patient to protect him from some harm does so in the context of a history and a relationship marked by many nondecisional elements, including the previous understandings between them, the motivations for judgment and action, and some degree of trust. The *decision* to lie is thus only a small part of "ethics" in this example. Assuming that their previous interactions were marked by honesty, the physician who lies to her patient changes their relationship and redefines herself. Surrounding her decision are deliberations, imaginings, and intentions that precede, inform, follow, and inevitably alter who this physician is, and who she is with and for this patient.

This complex, contextual background necessarily gives decisions in response to conventional moral dilemmas a larger meaning, because responding to moral dilemmas requires decision makers to identify, critically assess, and prioritize their moral values in order to find actions that express these values. Yet this is no simple matter, for three reasons. First, moral actors may be unsure just which commitments they want to express. Often our deepest convictions are not transparent to us, and we may have to work to discover them. Second, putting our convictions and commitments into practice requires many different capacities and skills. Ethics is part logic (following an argument), part leaps of imagination (stepping into someone else's shoes), part storytelling (weaving a coherent thread through our moral motives, means, and actions), and many other things. Ethics involves many faculties and capacities. It is not just a function of clear reasoning capacity or benevolent feelings, of having the right rules or principles, or of possessing good intentions or achieving good outcomes. Instead, ethics involves all of these human capacities in ways that require moral actors to understand that their whole selves are involved. Third, because ethical choices engage our most deeply held and self-defining expressions, no one terminology for describing ethics predominates. For example, in explaining the first two points above we have alternatively talked about "values," "commitments," and "convictions." This multifaceted language signals that ethics is more than aesthetic preferences or tastes, more than consumer-style choices or desires. Ethics is too large and important to be confined to one standard set of linguistic terms, and this variety can sometimes lead to confusion. We will return to this pluralism in ethical expression later in this essay, when considering ethical theories and the importance of an eclectic approach.

### Ethics as Human and Humanizing

Ethics appears to be distinctively human. Many other animals seem to be capable of moral behavior—shame, loyalty, helping others—and practice it routinely. But it is the capacity to systematically and critically reflect on one's moral behavior that seems to be uniquely characteristic of ethics. Ethics is not simply skill in doing good, but knowing *why* what one is doing can be called "good," having self-consciously chosen it from among the alternatives. As far as we can discern, only humans practice ethics in this reflective sense.

Ethics is also a *humanizing* activity. Conversations in ethics require viewing others with respect and regard; an exchange in ethics begins with the assumption that others are of value, and are subjects of a rich and complex life, just as we are. This simple gesture of respect is humanizing because it means that moral actors are willing to set aside, at least for the moment, differences in power and status in order to engage in ethics discussion with another.

This suspension of status and power enables attention to the other person—and, reflexively, also to oneself. Thus, engaging in ethical deliberation means listening—paying attention—and draws upon our empathic capacity. David Hume (1711–1776), Adam Smith (1723–1790), and other philosophers of the Scottish Enlightenment were the most systematic and sophisticated students of this capacity, which they termed "sympathy" or "fellow feeling" (Hume 1978; Smith 1976). The education and refinement of this universal capacity for empathy through reasoned reflection was for them the core of ethics. As Hume and Smith saw it, ethics could be said to be humanizing because it depends upon the further development, through reason and reflection, of a basic capacity that we seem to share with other animals.

Ethics requires us, and sympathy enables us, first to recognize other persons as sentient and reflective beings whose moral commitments are as important to them as our own values are to us, and then to vigorously and respectfully engage with others and their values. This engagement is not easy. Americans tend to be tolerant of differences and sometimes reluctant to discuss them. Often they fear disagreement and see it as counterproductive or polarizing, as if acknowledging divergence in moral convictions would make conversation difficult and consensus impossible. Yet this kind of tolerant reluctance can be as debilitating for ethics as is the hardened ideological positioning it seeks to avoid.

Genuine ethical inquiry arises from the rich human background we have been describing, and is characterized by openness to and exploration of differences. This "moral agnosticism" stands in opposition to moralizing or proselytizing for one's position, and also in opposition to the tolerant relativism that would avoid endorsing any position at all. It says, "I have strong convictions, but I also know that I alone do not possess the final truth." Such a demeanor seeks the best options through a careful examination of the ethical implications of all the possibilities, and a careful probing of the larger meaning of these options. The assumption that all parties engaged have a morally significant human voice (if not finally a fully persuasive position on resolving an issue) is the basic condition for dialogue. This assumption can also make consensus easier and the larger task of community building possible.

Engagement with others in moral discussion is humanizing in yet another way. The mutual empathy and respectful regard for differences that lets values emerge in an exchange is also a mode of interacting that is vastly less harmful for the participants. Anyone who has been involved in a situation that threatened to turn violent will immediately grasp the importance of this humanizing function. Ethics discussion can be thought of as a way of dealing with differences—one that is superior to many other modes of handling disagreements, such as shouting matches, holding grudges, filing lawsuits, or shooting people.

Perhaps most important, the assumption of the moral importance of multiple voices makes community possible both before and after decisions have been made. Because moral dialogue is a mode of mutual recognition and respect, it has a positive effect on human bonding and community building even when it fails as a mechanism of problem solving or consensus. Ethics has intrinsic value, not just instrumental value as a means to an end. It is sometimes said that virtue is its own reward. This means not only that the virtuous should not necessarily expect to become rich and famous but also that being virtuous teaches one a better set of rewards than money or fame: the benefits of integrity, compassion, and self-respect. Engaging others in moral dialogue inherently advances personal and communal life in ways that have little to do with decisions, outcomes, or consequences. Thus, while it may lead to better decisions and outcomes, ethics as an activity is also its own reward.

### Practicality, Expertise, and Common Moral Wisdom

Ethics is eminently practical. It is about how to live our lives, what choices to make, and ultimately who we are, individually and relationally. A number of moral theories and traditions commonly invoked in medical ethics are discussed later in this essay. For now it is important to note that theories and traditions often have practical utility, because they contain some portion of distilled wisdom about what is good or right. Yet theorizing is a means, not an end. An ethical theory or moral tradition that cannot provide usable moral guidance should be discarded as irrelevant. Whether a utilitarian approach is superior to a Kantian one, or whether libertarian perspectives are superior to communitarian ones, are unimportant questions standing alone. These theories have moral meaning only when we have a problem about which we are seeking guidance through them. The questions of ethics are always concrete and particular, and theoretical maneuvers must always be in the service of practical aims. For example, the question "Is the Kantian imperative to treat persons as 'ends in themselves' helpful for deciding whether to deceive this patient, at this time, for beneficent purposes?" asks whether a particular theoretical tool can help moral actors make a good moral choice in particular circumstances. To quote an old saw: "In theory, there's no difference between theory and practice. In practice, there is." Practical life is the testing ground for ethical theory, not vice versa.

Given its complexity and practical importance, ethics might be (indeed, has been) thought to be a field for experts. In the past, physicians, priests, and sometimes lawyers were thought to be the experts in medical ethics. In contemporary society, bioethicists and moral philosophers are often assigned that role. While there is a place for consulting authorities and moral expertise—and real benefit from studying Hippocrates, Aristotle, Kant, and Nietzsche, not to mention Freud, Jung, Gilligan, and dozens of others—the insights of these scholars and the traditions and theories they represent can be made accessible to anyone. A major task of ethical deliberation is determining just which parts of these traditions and theories are useful tools for moral discernment in particular cases. The practical skills of ethical discernment, reflection, and deliberation are available to everyone and, with some study, the tools of various traditions and theories can be available as well.

Ethical decisions can be very challenging, but what makes them challenging is not difficulty in mastering the writings of moral "experts." When ethical dialogue goes sour, or decisions go wrong, it is *not* because ethics as an activity requires highly specialized knowledge or theories intelligible only to a select few. When an ethical problem seems chronic or insoluble, it is often the case that insufficient attention has been paid to the dynamics of moral encounter: to the settings and relationships in which ethical problems develop. Maybe sometimes we do need more and better theories. Far more often, however, it is more helpful to seek better modes of human engagement—to create and maintain a "moral space" (Walker 1993) within which we may safely encounter ourselves and each other. Ethical discussions that become polarized are more often failures of the heart and the imagination than failures of the cortex.

The final aim of ethics is more than good decisions; it is a good life, a life marked by moral wisdom acquired through experience and reflection. Developing and consulting that reservoir of moral wisdom is a lifelong task. We are not morally transparent to ourselves; finding and critically affirming our values takes real work and the help of conversation partners. This was one of the most important lessons of Socrates. Moral traditions and theories can assist us in the work of locating, articulating, and testing the value-laden components of our experience—especially when they are thought of as tools, rather than as recipes for action or answer books.

### Moral Traditions and Ethical Theories: A Beginning Inventory of Tools

Thus, being an ethically literate person means knowing what tools are available, and being a good doctor means having a working acquaintance with the traditions and major theories that are likely to be helpful in the situations physicians typically face. In Western moral tradition, theories of ethics can be roughly grouped into two domains: principle and virtue. Principle-based theories of ethics are currently dominant, but virtue-oriented approaches were synonymous with ethics until roughly the European and North American Enlightenment period (18th century), and they still play an important role.

*Principle-based theories*: Reasoning through principles is very familiar in Western thought; it is quasi-mathematical in style, seeking to deduce right choices from the application of norms. Principle-based reasoning forms the basis of much of American law and public policy, and it has strongly influenced modern medical ethics. Many recent professional codes of ethics are composed of principles, and some of the legal principles underlying the Bill of Rights—freedom of speech, freedom of religion, liberty and privacy, due process, and equal protection of the laws—have become thoroughly identified with health care ethics as a result of their importance in defining the rights of patients. The triumvirate of particular principles that shape most discussions of medical ethics—autonomy, beneficence, and justice—has been the centerpiece of medical ethics theory for several decades (Beauchamp and Childress 1994).

The principle of autonomy, or more fully, respect for autonomy, is the principle most often associated with patients' rights. Respecting the autonomy of patients means according them self-determination by viewing their decisions and choices as valid; it means not interfering with them (the "negative" right to be left alone) unless their actions injure others; and it also means assisting them in the exercise of their autonomy (for example, by providing information about health care decisions).

In contrast, the principle of beneficence focuses on the duty of health care providers to act in the best interests of the patient. Beneficence, which entails both "doing no harm" and trying to do good, is generally seen by health care providers as the most important moral principle in health care. Many moral quandaries in health care present themselves as conflicts between the principles of autonomy and beneficence, which are often dichotomized, as typified, for example, by patients' desires for a course of action that is contrary to doctors' duty to protect their health. It is important to recognize, however, that a number of key concepts and issues in health care ethics—in particular, informed consent, truth telling, and confidentiality—combine and weigh considerations of respect for autonomy and duties of beneficence, and careful analysis will uncover the relationships between them. These principles are frequently better understood not as inevitably competing but as potentially complementary.

Justice is usually understood to mean fairness, and it introduces a wider social dimension to individual caregiver-patient relationships than those aspects emphasized by autonomy and beneficence. Justice sometimes means addressing questions about the distribution of health care resources, and what it means to do so equally or fairly. It sometimes means considering whether health care should have a role in remedying injustices, past or present. Justice also focuses on questions like whether health care is (or should be) a right, and what that might mean. Growing recognition of the limits of the financial and material resources that can be applied to meet health care needs has helped to bring the larger political and social dimensions of health care ethics into the forefront of discussion and concern. The meaning of justice in health care, both domestically and globally, is a central concern of that inquiry.

Many of the major moral theories that have been applied to medical ethics are principle-based. The "deontological" or duty-based moral theory of Immanuel Kant (1724–1804), which emphasizes treating persons as "ends in themselves," rather than as objects to be used only as means for achieving the ends of others, has been influential in medical ethics' understanding of the principle of autonomy (1985). Jeremy Bentham (1748–1832) and

John Stuart Mill (1806–1873) are the most important exponents of utilitarianism, in which right actions are those which result in the greatest good or welfare for the greatest number. Utilitarian theories consider beneficence to be central (but they also prescribe that actions which do not harm others should not be interfered with by society, thus establishing autonomy as a good). These two theories—Kantian deontology and utilitarianism—are the ones most often cited in health care ethics. They are generally viewed as being in opposition, but can be and often are combined as the basis of much law and public policy (Arras and Steinbock 1995).

*Virtue-oriented theories*: Virtue (or character) is very different from principle as a way of thinking about ethics. It is not quandary-focused and does not present a set of rules or norms to apply to a problem. Virtue theory looks at persons. Instead of taking a choice or decision as the unit of analysis, virtue-oriented approaches insist that morality is first and foremost about the moral actor. Instead of asking whether an action is consistent with a principle, such as "What decision does beneficence require?," virtue theorists are more likely to ask "What does it mean to be a trustworthy physician in this situation?," focusing on a character trait of the person. Health professionals' codes and statements of ethics are often cast in virtue language rather than, or in addition to, the language of principles (for example, "The nurse should be honest" instead of "The nurse should tell the truth"). Western virtue theory has Greek roots, with Aristotle's (384–322 BCE) ethics being the best-known exemplar.

The term "character" is often associated with virtue ethics approaches. It refers to the way a group of virtues creates a distinguishing feature of an individual moral actor, just as we speak of a character in a dramatic production. Patients often focus on virtue and character more than on principles; many religious traditions express their norms in virtue language, enjoining their adherents to lead lives characterized by "faith, hope, and love," or to "have compassion." And virtue-oriented character formation is the chief aim of much of the moral instruction that families seek to pass on to children. The familiar childhood moral instruction "Be good!" is virtue language. In part because of its familiarity and in part because it is more challenging to apply to problems—where modern medical ethics focuses its attention—virtue-oriented thinking has not been the dominant approach over the past 50 years. Yet its revival by philosophers like Alasdair MacIntyre (1984) has spawned a renewed interest in virtue approaches to medical ethics. Pellegrino and Thomasma, for example, have systematically explored those virtues they see as essential to medical practice: fidelity to trust, compassion, phronesis (practical wisdom), justice, fortitude, temperance, integrity, and self-effacement (1993).

Most people in their personal and professional lives mix the language of principles with the language of virtues. Most of us also mix moral theories together when we are addressing issues, testing their suitability for the problem at hand, rather than stuffing the problem into a box labeled "autonomy" or "utilitarianism" and cutting off the parts that won't fit. This almost instinctively eclectic approach to practical moral problem solving represents a problem only if one is in search of an all-encompassing and final theory of ethics. For the everyday business of moral reflection, dialogue, and problem solving, a broad pluralism of theories and traditions is beneficial, since it is open to new approaches and the rediscovery of forgotten ones. One such theoretical rediscovery is *casuistry*, an analytical method revived by Albert Jonsen and Stephen Toulmin from Catholic moral theology (1988). Casuistry means, simply, reasoning by cases. It employs cases—not principles or virtues—as the unit of moral analysis, and reaches judgments on a case-by-case basis, rather than attempting to apply or extract general rules. Casuistry is particularly attractive for health care ethics because clinical medicine is case-focused.

Another theoretical innovation in ethics comes from recognizing that cases inevitably involve the weaving of a narrative, and *narrative ethics* has recently emerged to name a way of doing ethics that focuses not just on the case but on the story (Hunter 1991). Stories have storytellers, principal and minor characters, relationships, dramatic structure, and history. Stories can also often be told from multiple viewpoints, employing frames of reference of varying sizes: family, institution, community, and society. Using a narrative theory of ethics emphasizes that "the facts" of a case are never neutral or standing alone; they must be seen in their context in order to be fully understood and appreciated. For example, the patient's history, as presented by the doctor according to the conventions of medicine, may be different in highly significant ways from the patient's story, told by the patient, even when the factual details of the patient's "chief complaint" are identical in both accounts. Casuistry and narrative ethics thus both provide new insights and approaches to moral analysis.

Another new cluster of moral theories, even more difficult to characterize, might be loosely called *difference ethics*. They challenge the definitive position of Western ethical theories and assert the superiority of moral traditions other than those derived from the Greeks, Western religious traditions, or the Enlightenment. Feminist theories of ethics, for example, champion an ethics of care, compassion, and relationship over a traditional ethics based on reason and justice. Other theories build upon cross-cultural differences, arguing, for example, that individual autonomy has no meaning in non-Western cultures, where family and community are central or where religious traditions are not focused on the individual self. Some theories of difference ethics go on to make a deeper critique of moral philosophy in general, by highlighting power and inequality as a central but undiscussed issue in moral relationships both individual and societal, and by bringing questions about the uses of power to the foreground. Though most often associated with feminist ethics, power analysis is common also to the search for an African American perspective on bioethics, and to inquiries about the relationship between ethics and ethnicity and culture (Pellegrino, Flack, and McManus 1992; Tong 1993). It also has visible roots in modern medical ethics. For example, the recognition of inequality of power and knowledge between patients and physicians formed the basis for the doctrine of informed consent as it developed in the 1950s and 1960s (Faden and Beauchamp with King 1986).

### Is There a Distinctive Medical Ethic?

It is noteworthy that physicians have not been satisfied to apply whatever moral standards were available from religion, political philosophy, or the common morality of society, but have from the beginning of Western medicine insisted on their own code of ethics. In asking whether there is anything that could be called a distinctive medical ethic, we are asking whether the work of physicians *should* be governed by a special ethic, a set of norms that are particular to doctors because of the work they do. The definition of medicine as a profession is linked to the idea that physicians are in some sense set apart by the nature of their work, destined for a different, if not higher, set of standards. They are, after all, asked to do some difficult things, such as train in relative social deprivation over long hours for many years, perform tasks in which their own health and safety may be at risk, and work in contexts that require patients to be extraordinarily vulnerable, both bodily and in terms of personal identity. Does this work require a set of standards that are, if not higher, at least somewhat more demanding?

Physicians since the Hippocratics have thought so. The Hippocratic oath not only describes the moral aspirations of a small sect of ancient Greek physicians but also invokes standards that set these physicians apart from other kinds of healers on moral/spiritual grounds. When this oath was first recited, it was a radical statement of highly stringent behavioral standards for a priestly brotherhood. So it appropriately begins with a pledge to "Apollo, Asclepius, Hygieia, Panaceia, and all the gods and goddesses." Today, appropriately sanitized of ancient Greek deities, the oath has come to be seen as stating many commonly held medical values. The various codes and statements of principle that physicians have put forward since the Hippocratic oath also serve as indices of medicine's dominant moral sensibility, indicating medicine's view of which issues are important and what standards should govern physicians' actions. Moreover, these codes are testimony to the need of physicians to state their standards publicly, as a way to signal to society that physicians are "worthy to serve the suffering" (the motto of Alpha Omega Alpha, the national medical honor society, as it appears on the title page of the journal *Pharos*).

Because physicians have thought of themselves as to some degree set apart for arduous and important work, graduating classes of doctors all over the United States typically recite an oath. Sometimes this is a revised version of the Hippocratic oath, with the pagan deities and some of the more problematic injunctions (such as the prohibition against using the knife) excised. For others the commencement ceremony includes an affirmation of moral commitments that is discussed and agreed upon by the graduating class itself, often including many of the Hippocratic restrictions (such as the duty to keep confidences), but adding norms that reflect contemporary problems, such as pledging to work for an inclusive system of health care coverage.

A small sample of historical and contemporary codes of ethics is included in this volume. The reader is invited to consider not only the implications of what is reflected and omitted in these various formulations, but also the implications of having a separate or special set of norms for doctors. Codes of medical ethics are not just individual action guides for physicians. They also serve an important function as an expression of the medical profession's contract with society, pledging trustworthy behavior in exchange for social trust and power. In this vein, it is useful to ask why such codes are always authored by physicians, rather than being collaborative products of medicine's dialogue with patients and the larger public. Also, since codes of medical ethics serve to frame therapeutic relationships, should there be a complementary list of moral expectations and responsibilities for being a patient? If so, would these merely address being a "good" individual patient while one is sick, or should they also address collective social responsibilities, such as the distribution of scarce medical resources?

Medical codes of ethics must be considered as one of the most important moral traditions available for medical ethics, simply because they have been passed forward for over 2,500 years. "Tradition" is a term that means literally to pass along, or hand over. Of course in the process of handing over, things change; this is how traditions stay vibrant and relevant to their times. The most basic ethical challenge for doctors and medical students is to recognize themselves as part of a long and complex moral tradition, with an obligation to reflect critically on what is being passed along, discarding what is no longer useful and creating new ways to articulate and embody what is as yet unknown and unsaid about moral life in medicine.

### Using Tools to Approach Problems: An Illustration

To stress that many traditions and theories are important to medical ethics is to eschew the vision of a single all-encompassing moral framework. The idea that morality could be finally and definitively secured by discovering and then following some monolithic theory is not just a philosopher's dream but a common human aspiration. A simple, unified theoretical basis for ethics that could eliminate the endless disputes and the vexing uncertainty of medical ethics decisions, unambiguously identifying what is good and right, would clearly be comforting. All candidates for such a unifying system in the past have proved to be procrustean beds. In Greek mythology, Procrustes, a son of Poseidon, forces his guests to fit themselves into his bed, by either stretching or cutting off their legs. Ethical theories that claim universal scope do similar damage, lopping off important facets of cases and situations in an effort to make them fit the preconceptions of theory and denying to moral agents the all-important exercise of their own particular moral perceptions and judgments.

In the absence of such theoretical unity, the task becomes one of using the wide range of tools and traditions skillfully. To illustrate how some of the tools we have described might be put to use, consider the following simplified case.

A 23-year old female is brought to the emergency department by ambulance following a motor vehicle crash. She is in hemorrhagic shock from a severe pelvic fracture requiring surgery, and is currently unconscious. She is a Jehovah's Witness and has signed a statement refusing blood products. Her husband is not a Jehovah's Witness and wants her to be given blood. The patient's parents are also present and insist that she would not want it. Her husband states that she signed the form refusing blood before the birth of her 10-month-old son, and that she would do anything to save her own life in order to care for her son.

Should this patient be given life-saving blood products, or not? This is the immediate question. In responding, we will focus on how moral traditions and theories help by bringing to prominence important facets of the situation and by posing questions to frame and shape our perspective. Here are some of the questions that would be emphasized in the various approaches we have discussed.

What would it mean to seek to treat this patient as an end in herself, and not just a means? Does the form she has signed constitute her autonomous choice, in this case made in advance of the actual situation? Would a utilitarian approach, emphasizing the greatest overall good, mean saving this patient's life in order to satisfy the needs of her son and husband, rather than her parents' assessment of her wishes? Which of the medical virtues is it important to enact here—fidelity to trust in respecting the patient's religious convictions? Or perhaps courage, in overriding her parents and doing everything to save this patient's life? (There are other possible manifestations of both trust and courage in this situation, too, some of which lead in different directions.) A feminist interpretation might highlight the power struggle between family members over a female patient, whereas a narrative approach would want to know who constructed this version of the problem, whose story it is that is being played out here. Can a better version of this problem be constructed? What would make it "better"—that it is a more accurate description of the ethical problems, or a more complete story, or that it might lead to a quicker or different resolution? These questions are illustrative, not definitive or exhaustive. Being skilled in ethics means knowing how to pick up the conversation and continue it.

Three points in summary. First, consulting a wide range of approaches can better equip moral actors to make decisions that they (and others) can live with over time, decisions that honor rather than suppress the complexity of both the issues and the relationships involved. Second, the key element in a good decision is making discerning judgments: surveying the available tools, selecting the right ones for the job, and using them with a modicum of skill. Having a wide range of tools is important; if one's only tool is a hammer, every problem may look like a nail.

But of course this analogy of selecting tools for a defined job, while helpful, is too simplistic and mechanical. As we have emphasized, sometimes just finding the decision point for action from within a complex web of persons, events, and relationships is a more challenging ethical task than reaching a decision. The hard work of ethics may not be what to decide, but discerning *how* to decide, or even realizing that no decision is called for. It is characteristic of different ethical theories that they provide us not only with differing ways to solve a problem, but also with differing definitions of the problem itself and divergent pathways for the exercise of moral agency, that is, different perceptions of the moral roles of the persons engaged in the decision. Finally, whatever decisional apparatus we adopt (or reject) brings with it relational commitments, both spoken and unspoken. Recognizing and naming the unspoken commitments is an important nondecisional aspect of ethics. It is also a necessary step in moral maturity and wisdom.

Third, ethical decisions are synchronic moments in larger diachronic histories; they are only slices of moral life. In spite of their high drama, and the great weight and consequence they may have, especially in life-and-death settings, individual decisions may not by themselves be definitive in shaping anyone's moral identity. Sometimes difficult decisions are a matter of doing the best one can in tragic situations, where all the options are bad ones. When clear choices do not appear, and satisfying resolutions seem unlikely, the challenge lies in choosing the "least worst" alternative and muddling through. In these cases, then, moral routines and habits take on considerable importance in shaping an ethical life or being a good doctor, because they make up the background of resources and relationships against which moral decisions are understood and made. Ultimately, ethics is about the shaping of moral identity and the development and application of moral wisdom throughout life. However urgently we need good decisions, good intentions, or good outcomes, none of those individual endpoints is truly achievable or sustainable apart from the larger effort of learning to live a good life. The models and tools of moral decision making serve that larger goal and are also served by it.

## Conclusion: Getting Grounded

Readers may view this rich moral landscape, featuring many languages and approaches to ethical problems, and many theories behind these approaches, with apprehension or delight at the possible paths before them. Recognition of the wide range of methods and approaches possible in ethics can be empowering for some, yet for others it may seem paralyzing: Without a universal, overriding ethical framework, what is there to keep us from becoming adrift in relativism?

The fear of moral relativism has been a nagging, but misunderstood, problem for Western ethics since before Plato (427–347 BCE). Relativism is the assumption that since there is no universal and timeless, agreed-upon standard for ethics, then there are no standards at all—everything must be up for grabs. The choice is conceived as between ethical certainty and the moral abyss.

Without offering a full discussion here, we submit that the practical moral pluralism described in this essay, which draws from many moral theories and traditions, does not lead to relativism. A plurality of resources is no more problematic for ethics than for other disciplines. There are competing theories in economics, psychiatry, mathematics, and physics—to name just a few—and shifting theoretical viewpoints over time in all these fields, yet no one assumes that because economists or physicists disagree among themselves, and sometimes combine theories and approaches, these fields are riddled with relativism. And so it is for ethics.

The best protection against both absolutist and relativistic interpretations of ethics lies in recognition that the whole of ethics is, after all, a human enterprise, with the effort of persons and their hard-won moral wisdom the only assurance we have for the integrity of the effort. Those who worry about relativism and become skeptical typically forget that the basic aim of ethics is not final answers, but practical guidance and continual moral learning from life's experiences and choices. The place we have to stand is not upon a universal foundation of eternal truth, but simply on the ground, on our own feet. There is no knock-down argument to refute the relativist or silence the skeptic. The answer lies in a commitment to use what we have to pursue that wisdom of which we are capable, and to do so honestly and persistently. Montaigne (1533–1592) put it with characteristic pungency: "We seek other conditions because we do not understand the use of our own, and we go outside ourselves because we do not know what it is like inside. Yet there is no use our mounting on stilts, for on stilts we must still walk on our own legs. And on the loftiest throne in the world we are still sitting only on our own rump" (Montaigne 1965).

At the beginning of this essay we noted that ethics is often conceived simplistically as a series of sharp-edged questions requiring either/or decisions. We have sought to make it clear that the responses given to such questions must be nested in a far larger context than is at first evident. The question "Should a physician lie to a patient when the lie promises patient benefit?" is meaningless without considering the role and place of truthfulness in a therapeutic encounter. Likewise, "Is it good to be candid about medical mistakes, and if so, whose good is served?" must be posed in the larger context of the need for personal and professional forgiveness (Arendt 1957), given that all physicians will make mistakes that cause harm. And "Should physicians ever assist their terminally ill patients in suicide?" resides within a larger inquiry about the meaning and purpose of medical care at the end of life. Ethics is personal and decisional because it is first social and relational. It inevitably entails probing into the larger meaning of choices and sounding the deeper reservoirs of our common human wisdom.

### References

Arendt, H. 1957. *The Human Condition.* Chicago: University of Chicago Press.

Aristotle. 1941. "Nicomachean Ethics." *The Basic Works of Aristotle.* New York: Random House.

Arras, J., and B. Steinbock, B. 1995. *Ethical Issues in Modern Medicine.* 4th ed. Mountain View, Calif.: Mayfield Publishing.

Beauchamp, T., and J. Childress. 1994. *Principles of Biomedical Ethics.* 4th ed. New York: Oxford University Press.

Faden, R., and T. Beauchamp, with N. King. 1986. *A History and Theory of Informed Consent.* New York: Oxford University Press.

Hume, D. 1978. *A Treatise of Human Nature, Book III.* 2nd ed. Edited by L. A. Selby-Bigge and P. H. Nidditch. Oxford: Clarendon Press.

Hunter, K. M. 1991. *Doctor's Stories: The Narrative Structure of Medical Knowledge.* Princeton, N.J.: Princeton University Press.

Jonsen, A., and S. Toulmin. 1988. *The Abuse of Casuistry.* Berkeley: University of California Press.

Kant, I. 1985. *Foundations of the Metaphysics of Morals.* Translated by L. W. Beck. New York: Macmillan.

MacIntyre, A. 1984. *After Virtue,* Notre Dame, Ind.: University of Notre Dame Press.

Mill, J. S. 1979. *Utilitarianism.* Edited by G. Sher. Indianapolis, Ind.: Hackett Publishing.

Montaigne, M. 1976. *The Complete Essays of Montaigne.* Translated by Donald Frame. Stanford, Calif.: Stanford University Press.

Pellegrino, E., and D. Thomasma. 1993. *The Virtues in Medical Practice*. New York: Oxford University Press.

Pellegrino, E., H. Flack, and D. McManus. 1992. *African-American Perspectives on Biomedical Ethics*. Washington, D.C.: Georgetown University Press.

Smith, A. 1976. *The Theory of Moral Sentiments*. Edited by D. Raphael and A. Macfie. Indianapolis, Ind.: Liberty Classics.

Tong, R. 1993. *Feminine and Feminist Ethics*. Belcourt, Calif.: Wadsworth Publishing.

Walker, M. U. 1993. "Keeping moral space open." *Hastings Center Report* 23, no. 2: 33–40.

# Historical and Contemporary Codes of Ethics: The Hippocratic Oath, Maimonides' Prayer, the Declaration of Geneva, and the AMA Principles of Medical Ethics

## Oath of Hippocrates
Sixth Century BCE—First Century CE

Assumed to have been written by Hippocrates, the oath exemplifies the Pythagorean school rather than Greek thought in general. The oath of Hippocrates is one of the earliest and most important statements on medical ethics. Estimates of its actual date of origin vary from the sixth century BCE to the first century CE. Not only has the oath provided the foundation for many succeeding medical oaths, for example, the Declaration of Geneva, but it is still administered by many medical schools to graduating medical students, either in its original form or in a slightly altered version.

I swear by Apollo Physician and Asclepius and Hygieia and Panaceia and all the gods and goddesses, making them my witnesses, that I will fulfil according to my ability and judgment this oath and this covenant:

To hold him who has taught me this art as equal to my parents and to live my life in partnership with him, and if he is in need of money to give him a share of mine, and to regard his offspring as equal to my brothers in male lineage and to teach them this art—if they desire to learn it—without fee and covenant; to give a share of precepts and oral instruction and all the other learning to my sons and to the sons of him who has instructed me and to pupils who have signed the covenant and have taken an oath according to the medical law, but to no one else.

---

* Ludwig Edelstein, "The Hippocratic Oath: Text, Translation and Interpretation," from *Bulletin of the History of Medicine*, Supplement 1, 3. © 1943. Reprinted with permission of The Johns Hopkins University Press.

I will apply dietetic measures for the benefit of the sick according to my ability and judgment; I will keep them from harm and injustice.

I will neither give a deadly drug to anybody if asked for it, nor will I make a suggestion to this effect. Similarly I will not give to a woman an abortive remedy. In purity and holiness I will guard my life and my art.

I will not use the knife, not even on sufferers from stone, but will withdraw in favor of such men as are engaged in this work.

Whatever houses I may visit, I will come for the benefit of the sick, remaining free of all intentional injustice, of all mischief, and in particular of sexual relations with both female and male persons, be they free or slaves.

What I may see or hear in the course of the treatment or even outside of the treatment in regard to the life of men, which on no account one must spread abroad, I will keep to myself holding such things shameful to be spoken about.

If I fulfil this oath and do not violate it, may it be granted to me to enjoy life and art, being honored with fame among all men for all time to come; if I transgress it and swear falsely, may the opposite of all this be my lot.

### Daily Prayer of a Physician ("Prayer of Moses Maimonides")
1793?

Almighty God, Thou has created the human body with infinite wisdom. Ten thousand times ten thousand organs hast Thou combined in it that act unceasingly and harmoniously to preserve the whole in all its beauty— the body which is the envelope of the immortal soul. They are ever acting in perfect order, agreement, and accord. Yet, when the frailty of matter or the unbridling of passions deranges this order or interrupts this accord, then forces clash and the body crumbles into the primal dust from which it came. Thou sendest to man diseases as beneficent messengers to foretell approaching danger and to urge him to avert it.

Thou has blest Thine earth, Thy rivers, and Thy mountains with healing substances; they enable Thy creatures to alleviate their sufferings and to heal their illnesses. Thou hast endowed man with the wisdom to relieve the suffering of his brother, to recognize his disorders, to extract the

---

* "Daily Prayer of a Physician," translated by Harry Friedenwald, from *Bulletin of the Johns Hopkins Hospital*, vol. 28, 260–261, 1917.

healing substances, to discover their powers, and to prepare and to apply them to suit every ill. In Thine Eternal Providence Thou hast chosen me to watch over the life and health of Thy creatures. I am now about to apply myself to the duties of my profession. Support me, Almighty God, in these great labors that they may benefit mankind, for without Thy help not even the least thing will succeed.

Inspire me with love for my art and for Thy creatures. Do not allow thirst for profit, ambition for renown and admiration, to interfere with my profession, for these are the enemies of truth and of love for mankind and they can lead astray in the great task of attending to the welfare of Thy creatures. Preserve the strength of my body and of my soul that they ever be ready to cheerfully help and support rich and poor, good and bad, enemy as well as friend. In the sufferer let me see only the human being. Illumine my mind that it recognize what presents itself and that it may comprehend what is absent or hidden. Let it not fail to see what is visible, but do not permit it to arrogate to itself the power to see what cannot be seen, for delicate and indefinite are the bounds of the great art of caring for the lives and health of Thy creatures. Let me never be absent-minded. May no strange thoughts divert my attention at the bedside of the sick, or disturb my mind in its silent labors, for great and sacred are the thoughtful deliberations required to preserve the lives and health of Thy creatures.

Grant that my patients have confidence in me and my art and follow my directions and my counsel. Remove from their midst all charlatans and the whole host of officious relatives and know-all nurses, cruel people who arrogantly frustrate the wisest purposes of our art and often lead Thy creatures to their death.

Should those who are wiser than I wish to improve and instruct me, let my soul gratefully follow their guidance; for vast is the extent of our art. Should conceited fools, however, censure me, then let love for my profession steel me against them, so that I remain steadfast without regard for age, for reputation, or for honor, because surrender would bring to Thy creatures sickness and death.

Imbue my soul with gentleness and calmness when older colleagues, proud of their age, wish to displace me or to scorn me or disdainfully to teach me. May even this be of advantage to me, for they know many things of which I am ignorant, but let not their arrogance give me pain. For they are old and old age is not master of the passions. I also hope to attain old age upon this earth, before Thee, Almighty God!

Let me be contented in everything except in the great science of my profession. Never allow the thought to arise in me that I have attained to sufficient knowledge, but vouchsafe to me the strength, the leisure, and the ambition ever to extend my knowledge. For art is great, but the mind of man is ever expanding.

Almighty God! Thou hast chosen me in Thy mercy to watch over the life and death of Thy creatures. I now apply myself to my profession. Support me in this great task so that it may benefit mankind, for without Thy help not even the least thing will succeed.

### Declaration of Geneva
### (World Medical Association)

At the time of being admitted as a member of the medical profession:

I solemnly pledge myself to consecrate my life to the service of humanity;

I will give to my teachers the respect and gratitude which is their due;

I will practice my profession with conscience and dignity;

The health of my patient will be my first consideration;

I will respect the secrets which are confided in me, even after the patient has died;

I will maintain, by all the means in my power, the honor and the noble traditions of the medical profession;

My colleagues will be my sisters and brothers;

I will not permit considerations of age, disease or disability, creed, ethnic origin, gender, nationality, political affiliation, race, sexual orientation, or social standing to intervene between my duty and my patient;

I will maintain the utmost respect for human life from its beginning even under threat, and I will not use my medical knowledge contrary to the laws of humanity.

I make these promises solemnly, freely and upon my honor.

---

* "Declaration of Geneva," adopted by the 2nd General Assembly of the World Medical Association, Geneva, Switzerland, September 1948, and amended by the 22nd World Medical Assembly, Sydney, Australia, August 1968, the 35th World Medical Assembly, Venice, Italy, October 1983, and the 46th WMA General Assembly, Stockholm, Sweden, September 1994.

### Principles of Medical Ethics

Preamble

The medical profession has long subscribed to a body of ethical statements developed primarily for the benefit of the patient. As a member of this profession, a physician must recognize responsibility to patients first and foremost, as well as to society, to other health professionals, and to self. The following Principles adopted by the American Medical Association are not laws, but standards of conduct which define the essentials of honorable behavior for the physician.

I. A physician shall be dedicated to providing competent medical care, with compassion and respect for human dignity and rights.

II. A physician shall uphold the standards of professionalism, be honest in all professional interactions, and strive to report physicians deficient in character or competence, or engaging in fraud or deception, to appropriate entities.

III. A physician shall respect the law and also recognize a responsibility to seek changes in those requirements which are contrary to the best interests of the patient.

IV. A physician shall respect the rights of patients, colleagues, and other health professionals, and shall safeguard patient confidences and privacy within the constraints of the law.

V. A physician shall continue to study, apply, and advance scientific knowledge, maintain a commitment to medical education, make relevant information available to patients, colleagues, and the public, obtain consultation, and use the talents of other health professionals when indicated.

VI. A physician shall, in the provision of appropriate patient care, except in emergencies, be free to choose whom to serve, with whom to associate, and the environment in which to provide medical care.

VII. A physician shall recognize a responsibility to participate in activities contributing to the improvement of the community and the betterment of public health.

VIII. A physician shall, while caring for a patient, regard responsibility to the patient as paramount.

IX. A physician shall support access to medical care for all people.

* "Principles of Medical Ethics," adopted by the American Medical Association House of Delegates June 17, 2001.

## Case Study: Please Don't Tell!

Leonard Fleck and Marcia Angell

The patient, Carlos R., was a twenty-one-year-old Hispanic male who had suffered gunshot wounds to the abdomen in gang violence. He was uninsured. His stay in the hospital was somewhat shorter than might have been expected, but otherwise unremarkable. It was felt that he could safely complete his recovery at home. Carlos admitted to his attending physician that he was HIV-positive, which was confirmed.

At discharge the attending physician recommended a daily home nursing visit for wound care. However, Medicaid would not fund this nursing visit because a caregiver lived in the home who could adequately provide this care, namely, the patient's twenty-two-year-old sister Consuela, who in fact was willing to accept this burden. Their mother had died almost ten years ago, and Consuela had been a mother to Carlos and their younger sister since then. Carlos had no objection to Consuela's providing this care, but he insisted absolutely that she was not to know his HIV status. He had always been on good terms with Consuela, but she did not know he was actively homosexual. His greatest fear, though, was that his father would learn of his homosexual orientation, which is generally looked upon with great disdain by Hispanics.

Would Carlos's physician be morally justified in breaching patient confidentiality on the grounds that he had a "duty to warn"?

### Commentary

Leonard Fleck

If there were a home health nurse to care for this patient, presumably there would be no reason to breach confidentiality since the expectation

Leonard Fleck and Marcia Angell, "Case Studies: Please Don't Tell!," from *Hastings Center Report*, vol. 21, 39–40. © 1991. Reprinted by permission of The Hastings Center and L. Fleck.

would be that she would follow universal precautions. Of course, universal precautions could be explained to the patient's sister. In an ideal world this would seem to be a satisfactory response that protects both Carlos's rights and Consuela's welfare. But the world is not ideal.

We know that health professionals, who surely ought to have the knowledge that would motivate them to take universal precautions seriously, often fail to take just such precautions. It is easy to imagine that Consuela could be equally casual or careless, especially when she had not been specifically warned that her brother was HIV-infected. Given this possibility, does the physician have a duty to warn that would justify breaching confidentiality? I shall argue that he may not breach confidentiality but he must be reasonably attentive to Consuela's safety. Ordinarily the conditions that must be met to invoke a duty to warn are: (1) an imminent threat of serious and irreversible harm, (2) no alternative to averting that threat other than this breach of confidentiality, and (3) proportionality between the harm averted by this breach of confidentiality and the harm associated with such a breach. In my judgment, none of these conditions are satisfactorily met.

No one doubts that becoming HIV-infected represents a serious and irreversible harm. But, in reality, is that threat imminent enough to justify breaching confidentiality? If we were talking about two individuals who were going to have sexual intercourse on repeated occasions, then the imminence condition would likely be met. But the patient's sister will be caring for his wound for only a week or two, and wound care does not by itself involve any exchange of body fluids. If we had 240 surgeons operating on 240 HIV-infected patients, and if each of those surgeons nicked himself while doing surgery, then the likelihood is that only one of them would become HIV-infected. Using this as a reference point, the likelihood of this young woman seroconverting if her intact skin comes into contact with the blood of this patient is very remote at best.

Moreover in this instance there are alternatives. A frank and serious discussion with Consuela about the need for universal precautions, plus monitored, thorough training in correct wound care, fulfills what I would regard as a reasonable duty to warn in these circumstances. Similar instructions ought to be given to Carlos so that he can monitor her performance. He can be reminded that this is a small price for protecting his confidentiality as well as his sister's health. It might also be necessary to provide gloves and other such equipment required to observe universal precautions.

We can imagine easily enough that there might be a lapse in conscientiousness on Consuela's part, that she might come into contact with his blood. But even if this were to happen, the likelihood of her seroconverting is remote at best. This is where proportionality between the harm averted by the breach and the harm associated with it comes in. For if confidentiality were breached and she were informed of his HIV status, this would likely have very serious consequences for Carlos. As a layperson with no professional duty to preserve confidentiality herself, Consuela might inform other family members, which could lead to his being ostracized from the family. And even if she kept the information confidential, she might be too afraid to provide the care for Carlos, who might then end up with no one to care for him.

The right to confidentiality is a right that can be freely waived. The physician could engage Carlos in a frank moral discussion aimed at persuading him that the reasonable and decent thing to do is to inform his sister of his HIV status. Perhaps the physician offers assurances that she would be able to keep that information in strict confidence. The patient agrees. Then what happens? It is easy to imagine that Consuela balks at caring for her brother, for fear of infection.

Medicaid would still refuse to pay for home nursing care because a caregiver would still be in the home, albeit a terrified caregiver. Consuela's response may not be rational, but it is certainly possible. If she were to react in this way it would be an easy "out" to say that it was Carlos who freely agreed to the release of the confidential information so now he'll just have to live with those consequences. But the matter is really more complex than that. At the very least the physician would have to apprise Carlos of the fact that his sister might divulge his HIV status to some number of other individuals. But if the physician impresses this possibility on Carlos vividly enough, Carlos might be even more reluctant to self-disclose his HIV status to Consuela. In that case the physician is morally obligated to respect that confidentiality.

#### Commentary
Marcia Angell

It would be wrong, I believe, to ask this young woman to undertake the nursing care of her brother and not inform her that he is HIV-infected.

The claim of a patient that a doctor hold his secrets in confidence is strong but not absolute. It can be overridden by stronger, competing claims. For example, a doctor would not agree to hold in confidence a diagnosis of rubella, if the patient were planning to be in the presence of a pregnant woman without warning her. Similarly, a doctor would be justified in acting on knowledge that a patient planned to commit a crime. Confidentiality should, of course, be honored when the secret is entirely personal, that is, when it could have no substantial impact on anyone else. On the other hand, when it would pose a major threat to others, the claim of confidentiality must be overridden. Difficulties arise when the competing claims are nearly equal in moral weight.

In this scenario, does Consuela have any claims on the doctor? I believe she does, and that her claims are very compelling. They stem, first, from her right to have information she might consider relevant to her decision to act as her brother's nurse, and, second, from the health care system's obligation to warn of a possible risk to her health. I would like to focus first on whether Consuela has a right to information apart from the question of whether there is in fact an appreciable risk. I believe that she has such a right, for three reasons.

First, there is an element of deception in *not* informing Consuela that her brother is HIV-infected. Most people in her situation would want to know if their "patient" were HIV-infected and would presume that they would be told if that were the case. (I suspect that a private nurse hired in a similar situation would expect to be told—and that she would be.) At some level, perhaps unconsciously, Consuela would assume that Carlos did not have HIV infection because no one said that he did. Thus, in keeping Carlos's secret, the doctor implicitly deceives Consuela—not a net moral gain, I think.

Second, Consuela has been impressed to provide nursing care in part because the health system is using her to avoid providing a service it would otherwise be responsible for. This fact, I believe, gives the health care system an additional obligation to her, which includes giving her all the information that might bear on her decision to accept this responsibility. It might be argued that the information about her brother's HIV infection is not relevant, but it is patronizing to make this assumption. She may for any number of reasons, quite apart from the risk of transmission, find it important to know that he is HIV-infected.

Finally, I can't help feeling that this young woman has already been exploited by her family and that the health care system should not collude in doing so again. We are told that since she was twelve, she has acted as "mother" to a brother only one year younger, presumably simply because she is female, since she is no more a mother than he is. Now she is being asked to be a nurse, as well as a mother, again presumably because she is female. In this context, concerns about the sensibilities of the father or about Carlos's fear of them are not very compelling, particularly when they are buttressed by stereotypes about Hispanic families. Furthermore, both his father and his sister will almost certainly learn the truth eventually.

What about the risk of transmission from Carlos to Consuela? Many would—wrongly, I believe—base their arguments solely on this question. Insofar as they did, they would have very little to go on. The truth is that no one knows what the risk would be to Consuela. To my knowledge, there have been no studies that would yield data on the point. Most likely the risk would be extremely small, particularly if there were no blood or pus in the wound, but it would be speculative to say how small. We do know that Consuela has no experience with universal precautions and could not be expected to use them diligently with her brother unless she had some sense of why she might be doing so. In any case, the doctor has no right to decide for this young woman that she should assume a risk, even if he believes it would be remote. That is for her to decide. The only judgment he has a right to make is whether *she* might consider the information that her brother is HIV-infected to be relevant to her decision to nurse him, and I think it is reasonable to assume she might.

There is, I believe, only one ethical way out of this dilemma. The doctor should strongly encourage Carlos to tell his sister that he is HIV-infected or offer to do it for him. She could be asked not to tell their father, and I would see no problem with this. I would have no hesitation in appealing to the fact that Carlos already owes Consuela a great deal. If Carlos insisted that his sister not be told, the doctor should see to it that his nursing needs are met in some other way. In sum, then, I believe the doctor should pass the dilemma to the patient: Carlos can decide to accept Consuela's generosity—in return for which he must tell her he is HIV-infected (or ask the doctor to tell her)—or he can decide not to tell her and do without her nursing care.

## Invasions
Perri Klass

Morning rounds in the hospital. We charge along, the resident leading the way, the interns following, the two medical students last, pushing the cart that holds the patients' charts. The resident pulls up in front of a patient's door, the interns stop as well, and we almost run them over with the chart cart. It's time to present the patient, a man who came into the hospital late last night. I did the workup—interviewed him, got his medical history, examined him, wrote a six-page note in his chart, and (at least in theory) spent a little while in the hospital library, reading up on his problems.

"You have sixty seconds, go!" says the resident, looking at his watch. I am of course thinking rebelliously that the interns take as long as they like with their presentations, that the resident himself is long-winded and full of pointless anecdotes—but at the same time I am swinging into my presentation, talking as fast as I can to remind my listeners that no time is being wasted, using the standard hospital turns of phrase. "Mr. Z. is a seventy-eight-year-old white male who presents with dysuria and intermittent hematuria of one week's duration." In other words, for the past week Mr. Z. has experienced pain with urination, and has occasionally passed blood. I rocket on, thinking only about getting through the presentation without being told off for taking too long, without being reprimanded for including nonessential items—or for leaving out crucial bits of data. Of course, fair is fair, my judgment about what is critical and what is not is very faulty. Should I include in this very short presentation (known as a "bullet") that Mr. Z. had gonorrhea five years ago? Well, yes, I decide, and include it in my sentence, beginning, "Pertinent past medical history

Perri Klass, "Invasions," from *A Not Entirely Benign Procedure.* © 1987 by Perri Klass and G. P. Putnam, Inc. Reprinted by permission of the Putnam Publishing Group.

includes . . ." I don't even have a second to remember how Mr. Z. told me about his gonorrhea, how he made me repeat the question three times last night, my supposedly casual question dropped in between "Have you ever been exposed to tuberculosis?" and "Have you traveled out of the country recently?"

"Five years ago?" The resident interrupts me. "When he was seventy-three? Well, good for him!"

Feeling almost guilty, I think of last night, of how Mr. Z.'s voice dropped to a whisper when he told me about the gonorrhea, how he then went on, as if he felt he had no choice, to explain that he had gone to a convention and "been with a hooker—excuse me, miss, no offense," and how he had then infected his wife, and so on. I am fairly used to this by now, the impulse people sometimes have to confide everything to the person examining them as they enter the hospital. I don't know whether they are frightened by suggestions of disease and mortality, or just accepting me as a medical professional and using me as a comfortable repository for secrets. I have had people tell me about their childhoods and the deaths of their relatives, about their jobs, about things I have needed to ask about and things that have no conceivable bearing on anything that concerns me.

In we charge to examine Mr. Z. The resident introduces himself and the other members of the team, and then he and the interns listen to Mr. Z.'s chest, feel his stomach. As they pull up Mr. Z.'s gown to examine his genitals, the resident says heartily, "Well now, I understand you had a little trouble with VD not so long ago." And immediately I feel like a traitor; I am sure that Mr. Z. is looking at me reproachfully. I have betrayed the secret he was so hesitant to trust me with.

I am aware that my scruples are ridiculous. It is possibly relevant that Mr. Z. had gonorrhea; it is certainly relevant to know how he was treated, whether he might have been reinfected. And in fact, when I make myself meet his eyes, he does not look nearly as distressed at being examined by three people and asked this question in a loud booming voice as he seemed last night with my would-be-tactful inquiries.

In fact, Mr. Z. is getting used to being in the hospital. And in the hospital, as a patient, you have no privacy. The privacy of your body is of necessity violated constantly by doctors and nurses (and the occasional medical student), and details about your physical condition are discussed by the people taking care of you. And your body is made to give up its secrets with a variety of sophisticated techniques, from blood tests to X-rays to biopsies—the whole point is to deny your body the privacy that pathological processes need in order to do their damage. Everything must be brought to light, exposed, analyzed, and noted in the chart. And all this is essential for medical care, and even the most modest patients are usually able to come to terms with it, exempting medical personnel from all the most basic rules of privacy and distance.

So much for the details of the patient's physical condition. But the same thing can happen to details of the patient's life. For the remainder of Mr. Z.'s hospital stay, my resident was fond of saying to other doctors, "Got a guy on our service, seventy-eight, got gonorrhea when he was seventy-three, from a showgirl. Pretty good, huh?" He wouldn't ever have said such a thing to Mr. Z.'s relatives, of course, or to any nondoctor. But when it came to his fellow doctors, he saw nothing wrong with it.

I remember another night, 4:00 A.M. in the hospital and I had finally gone to sleep after working-up a young woman with a bad case of stomach cramps and diarrhea. Gratefully, I climbed into the top bunk in the on-call room, leaving the bottom bunk for the intern, who might never get to bed, and who, if she did, would have to be ready to leap up at a moment's notice if there was an emergency. Me, I hoped that, emergency or not, I would be overlooked in the top bunk and allowed to sleep out the next two hours and fifty-five minutes in peace (I reserved five minutes to pull myself together before rounds). I lay down and closed my eyes, and something occurred to me. With typical medical student compulsiveness, I had done what is called a "mega-workup" on this patient, I had asked her every possible question about her history and conscientiously written down all her answers. And suddenly I realized that I had written in her chart careful details of all her drug use, cocaine, amphetamines, hallucinogens, all the things she had said she had once used but didn't anymore. She was about my age and had talked to me easily, cheerfully, once her pain was relatively under control, telling me she used to be really into this and that, but now she didn't even drink. And I had written all the details in her chart. I couldn't go to sleep, thinking about those sentences. There was no reason for them. There was no reason everyone had to know all this. There was no reason it had to be written in her official chart, available for legal subpoena. It was four in the morning and I was weary and by no means clear-headed; I began to fantasize one scenario after another in which my careless remarks in this woman's record cost her a job, got her thrown into jail, discredited her forever. And as I dragged myself out of the top bunk and out to the nurses' station to find her chart and cross out the offending sentences with such heavy black lines that they could never be read, I was conscious of an agreeable sense of self-sacrifice—here I was, smudging my immaculate mega-writeup to protect my patient. On rounds, I would say, "Some past drug use," if it seemed relevant.

Medical records are tricky items legally. Medical students are always being reminded to be discreet about what they write—the patient can demand to see the record, the records can be subpoenaed in a trial. Do not make jokes. If you think a serious mistake has been made, do not write that in the record—that is not for you to judge, and you will be providing ammunition for anyone trying to use the record against the hospital. And gradually, in fact, you learn a set of evasions and euphemisms with which doctors comment in charts on differences of opinion, misdiagnoses, and even errors. "Unfortunate complication of usually benign procedure." That kind of thing. The chart is a potential source of damage; damage to the patient, as I was afraid of doing, or damage to the hospital and the doctor.

Medical students and doctors have a reputation for crude humor; some is merely off-color, which comes naturally to people who deal all day with sick bodies. Other jokes can be more disturbing; I remember a patient whose cancer had destroyed her vocal cords so she could no longer talk. In taking her history from her daughter we happened to find out that she had once been a professional musician, singing and playing the piano in supper clubs. For the rest of her stay in the hospital, the resident always introduced her case, when discussing it with other doctors, by saying, "Do you know Mrs. Q.? She used to sing and play the piano—now she just plays the piano."

As you learn to become a doctor, there is a frequent sense of surprise, a feeling that you are not entitled to the kind of intrusion you are allowed into patients' lives. Without arguing, they permit you to examine them; it is impossible to imagine, when you do your very first physical exam, that someday you will walk in calmly and tell a man your grandfather's age to undress, and then examine him without thinking about it twice. You get used to it all, but every so often you find yourself marveling at the access you are allowed, at the way you are learning from the bodies, the stories, the lives and deaths of perfect strangers. They give up their privacy in exchange for some hope—sometimes strong, sometimes faint—of the alleviation of pain, the curing of disease. And gradually, with medical training, that feeling of amazement, that feeling that you are not entitled, scars over. You begin to identify more thoroughly with the medical profession—of course you are entitled to see everything and know everything; you're a doctor, aren't you? And as you accept this as your right, you move further from your patients, even as you penetrate more meticulously and more confidently into their lives.

## The Use of Force
### William Carlos Williams

They were new patients to me, all I had was the name, Olson. Please come down as soon as you can, my daughter is very sick.

When I arrived I was met by the mother, a big startled looking woman, very clean and apologetic who merely said, Is this the doctor? and let me in. In the back, she added. You must excuse us, doctor, we have her in the kitchen where it is warm. It is very damp here sometimes.

The child was fully dressed and sitting on her father's lap near the kitchen table. He tried to get up, but I motioned for him not to bother, took off my overcoat and started to look things over. I could see that they were all very nervous, eyeing me up and down distrustfully. As often, in such cases, they weren't telling me more than they had to, it was up to me to tell them; that's why they were spending three dollars on me.

The child was fairly eating me up with her cold, steady eyes, and no expression to her face whatever. She did not move and seemed, inwardly, quiet; an unusually attractive little thing, and as strong as a heifer in appearance. But her face was flushed, she was breathing rapidly, and I realized that she had a high fever. She had magnificent blonde hair, in profusion. One of those picture children often reproduced in advertising leaflets and the photogravure sections of the Sunday papers.

She's had a fever for three days, began the father and we don't know what it comes from. My wife has given her things, you know, like people do, but it don't do no good. And there's been a lot of sickness around. So we tho't you'd better look her over and tell us what is the matter.

As doctors often do I took a trial shot at it as a point of departure. Has she had a sore throat?

Both parents answered me together, No . . . No, she says her throat don't hurt her.

Does your throat hurt you? added the mother to the child. But the little girl's expression didn't change nor did she move her eyes from my face.

Have you looked?

I tried to, said the mother, but I couldn't see.

As it happens we had been having a number of cases of diphtheria in the school to which this child went during that month and we were all, quite apparently, thinking of that, though no one had as yet spoken of the thing.

Well, I said, suppose we take a look at the throat first. I smiled in my best professional manner and asking for the child's first name I said, come on, Mathilda, open your mouth and let's take a look at your throat.

Nothing doing.

Aw, come on, I coaxed, just open your mouth wide and let me take a look. Look, I said opening both hands wide, I haven't anything in my hands. Just open up and let me see.

Such a nice man, put in the mother. Look how kind he is to you. Come on, do what he tells you to. He won't hurt you.

At that I ground my teeth in disgust. If only they wouldn't use the word "hurt" I might be able to get somewhere. But I did not allow myself to be hurried or disturbed but speaking quietly and slowly I approached the child again.

As I moved my chair a little nearer suddenly with one catlike movement both her hands clawed instinctively for my eyes and she almost reached them too. In fact she knocked my glasses flying and they fell, though unbroken, several feet away from me on the kitchen floor.

Both the mother and father almost turned themselves inside out in embarrassment and apology. You bad girl, said the mother, taking her and shaking her by one arm. Look what you've done. The nice man . . .

For heaven's sake, I broke in. Don't call me a nice man to her. I'm here to look at her throat on the chance that she might have diphtheria and possibly die of it. But that's nothing to her. Look here, I said to the child, we're going to look at your throat. You're old enough to understand what I'm saying. Will you open it now by yourself or shall we have to open it for you?

Not a move. Even her expression hadn't changed. Her breaths however were coming faster and faster. Then the battle began. I had to do it. I had to have a throat culture for her own protection. But first I told the parents that it was entirely up to them. I explained the danger but said that

I would not insist on a throat examination so long as they would take the responsibility.

If you don't do what the doctor says you'll have to go to the hospital, the mother admonished her severely.

Oh yeah? I had to smile to myself. After all, I had already fallen in love with the savage brat, the parents were contemptible to me. In the ensuing struggle they grew more and more abject, crushed, exhausted while she surely rose to magnificent heights of insane fury of effort bred of her terror of me.

The father tried his best, and he was a big man but the fact that she was his daughter, his shame at her behavior and his dread of hurting her made him release her just at the critical moment several times when I had almost achieved success, till I wanted to kill him. But his dread also that she might have diphtheria made him tell me to go on, go on though he himself was almost fainting, while the mother moved back and forth behind us raising and lowering her hands in an agony of apprehension.

Put her in front of you on your lap, I ordered, and hold both her wrists.

But as soon as he did the child let out a scream. Don't, you're hurting me. Let go of my hands. Let them go I tell you. Then she shrieked terrifyingly, hysterically. Stop it! Stop it! You're killing me!

Do you think she can stand it, doctor! said the mother.

You get out, said the husband to his wife. Do you want her to die of diphtheria?

Come on now, hold her, I said.

Then I grasped the child's head with my left hand and tried to get the wooden tongue depressor between her teeth. She fought, with clenched teeth, desperately! But now I also had grown furious—at a child. I tried to hold myself down but I couldn't. I know how to expose a throat for inspection. And I did my best. When finally I got the wooden spatula behind the last teeth and just the point of it into the mouth cavity, she opened up for an instant but before I could see anything she came down again and gripping the wooden blade between her molars she reduced it to splinters before I could get it out again.

Aren't you ashamed, the mother yelled at her. Aren't you ashamed to act like that in front of the doctor?

Get me a smooth-handled spoon of some sort, I told the mother. We're going through with this. The child's mouth was already bleeding. Her tongue was cut and she was screaming in wild hysterical shrieks. Perhaps I should have desisted and come back in an hour or more. No doubt it would have been better. But I have seen at least two children lying dead in bed of neglect in such cases, and feeling that I must get a diagnosis now or never I went at it again. But the worst of it was that I too had got beyond reason. I could have torn the child apart in my own fury and enjoyed it. It was a pleasure to attack her. My face was burning with it.

The damned little brat must be protected against her own idiocy, one says to one's self at such times. Others must be protected against her. It is social necessity. And all these things are true. But a blind fury, a feeling of adult shame, bred of a longing for muscular release are the operatives. One goes on to the end.

In a final unreasoning assault I overpowered the child's neck and jaws. I forced the heavy silver spoon back of her teeth and down her throat till she gagged. And there it was—both tonsils covered with membrane. She had fought valiantly to keep me from knowing her secret. She had been hiding that sore throat for three days at least and lying to her parents in order to escape just such an outcome as this.

Now truly she *was* furious. She had been on the defensive before but now she attacked. Tried to get off her father's lap and fly at me while tears of defeat blinded her eyes.

## The Lie
Lawrence D. Grouse

Annie is from New Hampshire and came here to the foothills of the Blue
Ridge Mountains for the horse show. The nurses and I carry her from the
car into the emergency room and gently place her on the gurney. She was
kicked in the abdomen by her horse and lay in a field for over an hour until
friends found her and brought her to the hospital. Even though I am working in the emergency room of a small hospital, I am confident. The nurses
know their jobs. Faced with a serious surgical problem, we work well
together.

Within a few minutes we have inserted two IVs, one in a forearm vein,
another in the external jugular; her blood pressure, however, remains mar-
ginal. The fluid from the abdominal tap is grossly bloody, and so is her
urine. Annie remains calm. Her serious eyes are piercing; I hold her hand
to reassure her, but also take her pulse. She is bleeding very rapidly into
her abdomen. Nothing I do seems to help, and I am scared. She is in shock,
yet she converses politely and inquires about her condition.

"Thank you for helping me," she says. "Really, it wasn't the horse's
fault!"

"We're not worried about the horse, Annie," I say. "The horse is fine."

"Is it a serious injury?" She pauses. "Will I live?"

"Everything will work out, Annie," I tell her. "It may be a little rough for
a bit, but it will work out."

"Are you sure?" she asks, gazing steadily at me. "Please, tell me honestly."

I don't answer for a moment. I look at her. I am already fond of her and

Lawrence D. Grouse, "The Lie," from *Archives of Internal Medicine*, vol. 157, 2153. © 1997 by
the American Medical Association. Reprinted by permission of the publisher.

I do not want to lie. I squeeze her hand and smile. I am unsure how she will do, but I say, "Yes, I'm sure."

After a third iv is in place, her blood pressure stabilizes. The general surgeon and the urologist arrive and plan their emergency workup and exploratory surgery. I breathe a sigh of relief as they take charge of her care. Suddenly, we find that the door to the surgical suite in the emergency room has been inadvertently locked and the head nurse's key won't open it. Annie and a nurse are locked inside. There is a great deal of key rattling and doorknob shaking. The pitch of people's voices starts to rise. I break into a sweat. The head nurse yells orders into the telephone and almost immediately three burly maintenance men with crowbars appear.

"Get rid of that door! Now!" the head nurse bellows.

The door is splintered in 20 seconds. Annie is laughing, tells us not to worry, tells us that she is fine. She thinks it is the funniest scene ever.

At surgery, we find that Annie has a severely lacerated liver and a ruptured kidney. The liver is repaired; the kidney is removed, but when I wake up the next morning and look in on Annie, disseminated intravascular coagulation has developed and she is receiving heparin. Four nurses and two physicians have already given blood for her. The intensive care unit hosts a steady stream of staff who have helped Annie and who come by with a few encouraging words. Her parents have arrived. Annie's father is a college professor: a tall, angular man, feeling frightened and out of place. Annie's mother is a small woman with delicate features. The surgeon's wife accompanies them. By the following day, when I leave the hospital after my weekend shift, several of the staff, including the head nurse, have each given two units of blood for Annie.

Two weeks later—during my next shift—I am waylaid and hugged by a happy and ambulatory Annie.

"Everyone here has been so good to me," Annie beams.

As we sit over a cup of coffee, her parents timidly inquire whether Annie might have been close to death on her arrival at the hospital. I can't help bragging about treating Annie in the emergency room. As I launch into the story, I find that Annie remembers it all, and she chimes in with an exact rendition of our entire conversation on the day of the accident. I am amazed! She was in shock, and still she remembers every word I said. I finish my story with a flourish. "When I found that you had abdominal bleeding and I still couldn't bring up your blood pressure with two ivs, I have to admit that I thought you were a goner."

Annie seems shocked to hear this. She looks at me angrily and says, "Don't you remember? You said you were sure I would live. I remembered that promise all the time! I put a great deal of weight on what you said, and you . . . ." Suddenly, for the first time since the accident, and to everyone's surprise, tears are in her eyes and she is weeping; she is inconsolable because I lied to her.

# Informed Consent, Cancer, and Truth in Prognosis
## George J. Annas

Barbara Tuchman records that during the Black Death epidemic in the early 14th century, "doctors were admired, lawyers universally hated and mistrusted."[1] The great plagues and wars of the Middle Ages produced a "cult of death," including a vast popular literature that had death as its theme. As the 20th century closes, our emphasis is on the denial of death, and the honest discussion of death remains rare both in popular literature and in conversations between physicians and patients. This is one reason why Shana Alexander shocked a national conference of bioethicists last year by saying, "I trust my lawyer more than I trust my doctor." What she meant, she explained, was that she trusted her lawyer to tell her the truth about her alternatives and to execute faithfully the one she chose; she did not have this confidence in her physician, at least not if she were critically ill.

To the extent that Alexander's attitude is shared by Americans, it is an indictment, because nowhere in medicine is trust so necessary as in physician-patient conversations near death. The national survey conducted by Louis Harris for a presidential commission on bioethics in 1982 supports her view. It found that 96 percent of Americans wanted to be told if they had cancer, and 85 percent wanted a "realistic estimate" of how long they had to live if their type of cancer "usually leads to death in less than a year."[2] On the other hand, fewer than half the physicians surveyed said they would either give a "straight statistical prognosis" (13 percent) or "say that you can't tell how long [the patient] might live, but stress that in most cases people live no longer than a year" (28 percent) if the patient had a "fully confirmed diagnosis of lung cancer in an advanced stage."[2]

The country's most recent important case involving informed consent, *Arato v. Avedon*,[3] centers on whether the law should require physicians to report statistical life-expectancy data to their patients in cases of illness that is likely to be terminal.

### The Case of Miklos Arato

On July 21, 1980, Miklos Arato, a 43-year-old electrical contractor, was operated on to remove a nonfunctioning kidney. During surgery a tumor was found in the tail of his pancreas, and the tumor, along with the surrounding tissue and lymph nodes, was removed. Several days later, the surgeon met with Mr. Arato and his wife. He told them that he thought he had removed all of the tumor and referred them to an oncologist. The surgeon did not tell them that only about 5 percent of patients with pancreatic cancer survive for five years or give Mr. Arato either a prognosis or a reasonable estimate of his life expectancy. The oncologist told the Aratos that there was a substantial chance of a recurrence, and that a recurrence would mean that the disease was incurable. He recommended experimental chemotherapy and radiation treatment, acknowledging that this might produce no benefit. The oncologist was not asked for and did not volunteer a prognosis.

While the chemotherapy and radiation treatment were continuing, on April 22, 1981, a recurrence was detected. Even though the physicians believed Mr. Arato's life expectancy could then be measured in months, they did not tell him so. Mr. Arato died on July 25, 1981, approximately one year after his cancer had been diagnosed. After his death, his wife and two adult children brought suit against the surgeons and oncologists, alleging that they had had an obligation, under California's informed-consent doctrine, to tell Mr. Arato, before asking him to consent to chemotherapy, that approximately 95 percent of people with pancreatic cancer die within five years.

### The Proceedings in the Lower Court

At trial it was shown that at the first meeting with his oncologist, Mr. Arato had filled out an 18-page questionnaire in which he answered "yes" to the question, "If you are seriously ill now or in the future, do you want to be told the truth about it?"[3] The physicians who treated Mr. Arato justified their nondisclosure of the statistical prognosis on a variety of grounds, most based on traditional medical paternalism. His surgeon, for example, thought Mr. Arato had shown such great anxiety about his cancer that it was "medically inappropriate" to disclose specific mortality rates. The chief oncologist said he understood that patients like Mr. Arato "wanted to be told, but did not want a cold shower." He thought that reporting extremely high mortality rates might "deprive a patient of any hope of a cure," and that this was medically inadvisable. His physicians also said that during his 70 visits with them over a one-year period, Mr. Arato had avoided ever specifically asking about his own life expectancy and that this indicated that he did not want to know the information. In addition, all the physicians testified that the statistical life expectancy of a group of patients had little predictive value when applied to a particular patient.[3,4]

Mrs. Arato argued that the statistical prognosis should have been disclosed because it indicated that even with successful treatment (the physicians measured success in terms of added months of survival), Mr. Arato would probably live only a short time. If Mr. Arato had known the facts, she believed, he would not have undergone the rigors of the experimental treatment, but would instead have chosen to live out his final days at peace with his wife and family and would have made final arrangements for his business affairs. Mr. Arato had failed to order his financial affairs properly before his death, which had resulted in the eventual failure of his contracting business and substantial tax losses after his death.

On the basis of standard California jury instructions on informed-consent requirements, the jury returned a verdict in favor of the physicians. The Aratos appealed. A California court of appeals reversed the decision in a two-to-one opinion, stating that physicians were under an obligation to disclose statistics concerning life expectancy to patients so that they might take timely action to plan for their deaths, including the financial aspects of their deaths.[4] The physicians then appealed.

### The California Supreme Court

The California Supreme Court unanimously reversed the appeals court's decision. The justices began their analysis by reviewing their own most important previous cases related to informed consent: *Cobbs v. Grant*,[5]

*Truman v. Thomas*,[6] and *Moore v. Regents of the University of California*.[7] The court noted, as it had in *Cobbs*, that the doctrine of informed consent is "anchored" in four postulates:

—patients are generally ignorant of medicine;
—patients have a right to control their own body and thus to decide about medical treatment;
—to be effective, consent to treatment must be informed;
—patients are dependent upon their physicians for truthful information and must trust them (making the doctor-patient relationship a "fiduciary" or trust relationship rather than an arms-length business relationship).[5]

In *Truman*, a case about the refusal of a patient to have a Pap smear, the court decided that information had to be disclosed even if the patient refused treatment "so that patients might meaningfully exercise their right to make decisions about their own bodies."[6] And in *Moore*, a case about creating an immortal cell line from a diseased spleen, the court held that the physician must disclose "personal interests unrelated to the patient's health, whether research or economic, that may affect the physician's personal judgment."[7] Instead of taking the opportunity to resolve what the California Supreme Court described as a "critical standoff" in the development of the doctrine of informed consent between the extremes of absolute patient sovereignty and medical paternalism, the court focused on one very narrow question: whether California's standard instructions to juries should be revised to require the specific disclosure of a patient's life expectancy as predicted by mortality statistics.[3]

Framing the question so narrowly made answering it relatively easy. The court described the physician-patient relationship as "an intimate and irreducibly judgment-laden one" that had to be judged within "the overall medical context."[3] As for statistics on life expectancy, the court found them of little use to individual patients. The court thought, for example, that "statistical morbidity values derived from the experience of population groups are inherently unreliable and offer little assurance regarding the fate of the individual patient."[3]

Perhaps most important, the court described this case as one that was "fairly litigated" and properly put in the hands of "the venerable American jury," which had rendered a reasonable verdict that it was not prepared to second-guess.[3] The court concluded:

Rather than mandate the disclosure of specific information as a matter of law, the better rule is to instruct the jury that a physician is under a legal duty to disclose to the patient all material information—that is, information which would be regarded as significant by a reasonable person in the patient's position when deciding to accept or reject a recommended medical procedure—needed to make an informed decision regarding a proposed treatment.[3]

The patient's desire to be told the truth, as evidenced by his answer on the questionnaire, was found to be irrelevant, since the physician has an independent legal duty to tell the "truth" (although a patient can waive the right to information). The court also dealt with the issue of expert testimony, noting that in addition to the information required to be disclosed by *Cobbs*[5] (the nature and benefits of the proposed treatment, its risks of death or serious harm, reasonable alternatives and their risks, and problems of recuperation), physicians must also disclose any other information that another skilled practitioner would disclose. The court ruled that specific data on life expectancy fell within this standard. Thus, the defendant physicians were properly permitted to call expert medical witnesses to testify that it was not standard practice in the medical community in 1980 to disclose specific life-expectancy data.

### Prognosis and Success

If the only issue is whether the law should require physicians always to disclose statistical life-expectancy data to critically ill patients as part of the informed-consent process, the conclusion of the court is defensible. But this is much too narrow a basis for the decision. Although by itself the statistical probability of survival for an individual patient may not be material, it is material if it indicates whether the patient is likely to survive and the probable quality of life with and without treatment. In other words, the issue of informed consent in this instance centers on the disclosure of the success rate of the proposed treatment in terms of both the prospects for long-term survival and the patient's quality of life. This is what patients need to know, and this is the type of material information patients have a right to—not only because it is the patient's body, but, more important, because it is the patient's life.[8]

It is unfortunate that the plaintiff did not argue the case on the grounds of the necessity to explain success rates, because the results could have (and should have) been different. In *Cobbs*, which *Arato* affirms, the California Supreme Court had said:

> A medical doctor, being the expert, appreciates the risks inherent in the procedure he is prescribing, the risks of a decision not to undergo the treatment, and the probability of a successful outcome of the treatment. . . . The weighing of these risks against the individual subjective fears and hopes of the patient is not an expert skill. Such evaluation and decision is a nonmedical judgment reserved to the patient alone.[5]

This language explicitly requires physicians to explain the probability that a proposed treatment will be successful and implicitly requires the physician to tell the patient what the physician means by "success."[9] In this case, for example, the court seems correct in concluding that a statistical life-expectancy profile of all patients with pancreatic cancer, by itself, might not have been required to inform Mr. Arato of his prognosis properly. But such information is very valuable when coupled with an explanation of why the physician thinks the patient's case is or is not typical. Group data are the basis for predictions in individual cases—including both treatment recommendations and statements about probable risks and benefits. The physicians relied on group data, for example, to tell Mr. Arato that if his cancer recurred it would be "incurable." The court should have made it clearer that it is always material to a reasonable person to know both the probability of success of a proposed treatment and the meaning of success. Without this information, it is the physician, not the patient, who is making the treatment decision, and that is precisely what the doctrine of informed consent is designed to prevent.

### Culture and Death

A culture's general attitude toward death strongly influences what information about their prognosis will be provided to terminally ill patients. In the Middle Ages, for example, "when death was to be met any day around the corner, it might have been expected to become banal; instead it exerted a ghoulish fascination."[1] There was an emphasis on "worms and putrefaction and gruesome physical details"; instead of emphasizing a spiritual journey, the culture concentrated on the rotting of the body.[1] In our culture, with its unprecedented life expectancy, we tend to deny death altogether and celebrate new forms of medical technology designed to forestall death. In this context, it is not surprising that physicians often conceal prognostic information from their patients, just as most physicians once refused to use the word "cancer."[9] But concealment of prognosis from patients near death makes them feel abandoned and makes physicians feel estranged.[10,11] Candor toward the dying is an old problem, which Tolstoy described so well in "The Death of Ivan Ilych": "What tormented Ivan Ilych most was the deception, the lie . . . that he was not dying but was simply ill, and that he only need keep quiet and undergo treatment and then something very good would result."[12]

Ilych, a former prosecutor, also recognized that his physician's manner, which implied "if only you put yourself in our hands we will arrange everything—we know indubitably how it has to be done, always the same way for everybody alike," was "just the same air towards him as he himself put on towards an accused person."[12] Of course, the doctrine of informed consent is based on the recognition that people are not all the same and that physicians must let patients decide about treatment options so that they do not treat them "always the same way for everybody alike." In the treatment of cancer, the problem is especially acute because it is complicated by the financial conflicts of interest of oncologists. The chief beneficiaries of unproved cancer treatments are often the "appointment book of the oncologist" and "the pharmaceutical companies and their stockholders."[13] It is also likely that there would be far less aggressive treatment at the end of life if patients were honestly informed of the "sheer futility" of such experimental interventions.[13]

After more than two decades of legal and ethical debate, neither the idea nor the ideal of informed consent governs the doctor-patient relationship.[9,10,11,13] Jay Katz has properly noted that for conditions in which "prognosis is dire and fatal outcome a likely prospect . . . physicians should be guided by the strongest presumption in favor of disclosure and consent which can be modified only by clear and carefully documented evidence that patients do not wish to be fully informed."[14] In affirming *Cobbs*, the court's decision in *Arato*, although very narrow, is consistent with Katz's vision and should be understood as an affirmation of information sharing and patient-centered decision making in the context of a physician-patient relationship based on trust.

## Notes

1  Tuchman, B.W. A distant mirror: the calamitous 14th century. New York: Ballantine Books, 1978:58.

2  President's Commission for the Study of Ethical Problems in Medicine and Biomedical and Behavioral Research. Making health care decisions: the ethical and legal implications of informed consent in the patient-practitioner relationship. Vol. 2. Appendices. Washington, D.C.: Government Printing Office, 1982:245–6.

3  Arato v. Avedon, 5 Cal. 4th 1172, 23 Cal. Rptr.2d 131, 858 P.2d 598 (1993).

4  Arato v. Avedon, 13 Cal. App. 4th 1325, 11 Cal. Rptr.2d 169 (1992).

5  Cobbs v. Grant, 8 Cal.3d 229, 104 Cal. Rptr. 505, 502 P.2d 1 (1972).

6  Truman v. Thomas, 27 Cal.3d 285, 165 Cal. Rptr. 308, 611 P.2d 902 (1980).

7  Moore v. Regents of the University of California, 51 Cal.3d 120, 271 Cal. Rptr. 146, 793 P.2d 479 (1990).

8  Capron, A.M. Duty, truth, and whole human beings. Hastings Cent Rep 1993;23(4):13–4.

9  Annas, G.J. The rights of patients: the basic ACLU guide to patient rights. 2nd ed. Carbondale: Southern Illinois University Press, 1989.

10  Cassel, C.K., Meier, D.E. Morals and moralism in the debate over euthanasia and assisted suicide. N Engl J Med 1990;323:750–2.

11  Katz, J. The silent world of doctor and patient. New York: Free Press, 1984.

12  Tolstoy, L. The death of Ivan Ilych. New York: New American Library, 1960.

13  Moertel, C.G. Off-label drug use for cancer therapy and national health care priorities. JAMA 1991;266:3031–2.

14  Katz, J. Physician-patient encounters "On a darkling plain." W N Engl Law Rev 1987;9: 207–26.

# Offering Truth: One Ethical Approach to the Uninformed Cancer Patient

Benjamin Freedman

Medical and social attitudes toward cancer have evolved rapidly during the last 20 years, particularly in North America.[1,2] Most physicians, most of the time, in most hospitals, accept the ethical proposition that patients are entitled to know their diagnosis. However, there remains in my experience a significant minority of cases in which patients are never informed that they have cancer or, although informed of the diagnosis, are not informed when disease progresses toward a terminal phase. Although concealment of diagnosis can certainly occur in cases of other terminal or even nonterminal serious illnesses, it seems to occur more frequently and in more exacerbated form with cancer because of the traditional and cultural resonances of dread associated with cancer.

These cases challenge our understanding of and commitment to an ethical physician-patient relationship. In addition, they are observably a significant source of tension between health care providers. When the responsible physician persists in efforts to conceal the truth from patients, consultant physicians, nurses, social workers, or others may believe that they cannot discharge their functions responsibly until the patient has been told. Alternatively, when a treating physician decides to inform the patient of his or her diagnosis, strong resistance from family members who have instigated a conspiracy of silence may be anticipated.

This essay outlines one approach, employed in my own ethical consultations and at some palliative care services or specialized oncology units. This approach, offering truth to patients with cancer, affords a means of satisfying legal and ethical norms of patient autonomy, ameliorating conflicts between families and physicians, and acknowledging the cultural norms that underlie family desires.

### Common Features of Cases

Mrs. A. is a woman in her 60s with colon cancer, with metastatic liver involvement and a mass in the abdomen. She is not expected to survive longer than weeks. Other than a course of antibiotics, which she was just about to complete, no active treatment is indicated or intended. She is alert. She knows that she has an infection; her family refuses to inform her that she has cancer. The precipitating cause of the ethical consultation, requested by the newly assigned treating physician (Dr. H.), is his ethical discomfort with treating Mrs. A. in this manner.

When one is confronted with a case of concealment, it is worth wondering how it came about that everyone but the patient has been told of the diagnosis, so that similar situations may be avoided in the future. Often, a diagnosis is defined in the course of surgery and disclosed to waiting relatives; this may most appropriately be handled by a prior understanding with the patient, communicated to the family, as to whether and how much they will be told before the patient awakens. But there are at least two other major ways in which a situation of concealment might develop.

A patient might be admitted in medical crisis, at a time when he or she is obtunded and incapable of being informed of his or her condition and treatment options. Law and ethics alike require that the medical team inform and otherwise deal with the person who is most qualified to speak on the patient's behalf (usually, the next of kin), until the patient has recovered enough to speak for himself or herself. Unfortunately for this plan, though, a patient will often fail to cross, at one moment, the bright line from incompetent to competent. Consequently, patterns of communicating with the relative instead of with the patient may persist beyond the intended period. Such situations have their own momentum. Later disclosure to the patient will need to deal both with the burden of providing bad news and with the fact that this information has been concealed from the patient up to that point.

A second typical way in which concealment develops is the following. A patient with close family ties is always attended by a relative (commonly, spouse or child) at medical appointments. Before a firm diagnosis is established, that relative manages to elicit a promise from the physician not to tell the patient should the tests show that the patient has cancer. Faced with a distraught and deeply caring relative, the physician goes along, at least as a temporizing tactic, only to discover, as described above, how the situation develops its own inertia. The cycle may be broken in a number of ways. Sometimes the physician simply decides to call a halt to concealment; often the patient's care is transferred to another physician who has not been a party to the conspiracy, as had happened with Mrs. A.

> As clinical ethicist, I met with Dr. H. and the relevant family members (husband, daughter, and son). Most of the discussion was held with the son; the husband, a first-generation Greek-Canadian immigrant, knows little English and was at any rate somewhat withdrawn. As expected, they are a close family, deeply solicitous of the patient, and convinced that she will suffer horribly were she to be told she has cancer. They confirmed my sense that the Greek cultural significance of cancer equals death—something that in this case is in all likelihood true.
>
> At this time the family was willing to sign any document we wanted them to, assuming all responsibility for the decision to conceal the truth from Mrs. A. "Do us this one favor" was a plea that punctuated the discussion.

Although other factors, such as the context of treatment and the patient's own idiosyncratic personality, may cause the same kind of problem in communication, my experience suggests the situation is often, as here, mediated by cultural factors. As one text on ethnic factors in family counseling puts it, "Greek Americans do not believe that the truth shall make you free, and the therapist should not attempt to impose the love of truth upon them."[3] (And compare Dalla-Vorgia et al.[4]) I often find other immigrant families of Mediterranean or Near Eastern origin reacting similarly, for example, Italian families and those of Sephardic Jews who have immigrated from Morocco. In all cases, in my experience, there is a special plea on the part of families to respect their cultural pattern and tradition. Health care providers often feel the force of this claim and its corollary: informing the patient would be an act of ethical and cultural imperialism. Moreover, the family not uncommonly feels strongly enough that legal action is threatened unless their wishes are respected. Mrs. A.'s family, in fact, threatened to sue at one point when they were told that Mrs. A.'s diagnosis would be revealed.

By the time a clinical ethical consultation is requested, the situation has often become highly charged emotionally. In addition to the unpleasantness of threats of legal action, there may have been some physical confrontation.

> Mrs. S. was a Sephardic woman in her 70s with widespread metastatic seedings in the pleura and pericardium from an unknown primary tumor. Her family insisted that she not be informed of her diagnosis and prognosis. Suffering from a subjective experience of apnea, she was to have a morphine drip begun to alleviate her symptoms. The family physically expelled the nurse from the room. If their mother were to learn she was getting morphine, they said, she would deduce that her situation was grave.

Such aberrant behavior cannot fairly be understood without realizing that these families may be acting out of uncommonly deep concern for the well-being of the patient, as they (perhaps misguidedly) understand it. The health care team shares the same ultimate goal, to care for the patient in a humane, decent, caring manner. This commonality can serve as the basis for continuing discussion, as in the above case of Mrs. A., the Greek patient.

> Discussion with the family was long and meandering. The usual position of the health care team was explained in some detail: patients in our institution are generally told their diagnosis; we are accustomed to telling patients that they have cancer, and we know how to handle the varied normal patient reactions to this bad news; patients do not (generally) kill themselves immediately on being told, or die a voodoo death, in spite of the family's fears and cultural beliefs about patient reaction to this diagnosis. Patients have a right to this information and may have the need to attend to any number of tasks pending death: to say good-bye, to make arrangements, to complete unfinished business. As her illness progresses, decisions will likely need to be made about further treatment, for example, of infections or blockages that develop. Already, one of Mrs. A.'s kidneys is blocked and her urine is backing up. If the mass should obstruct her other kidney, for example, should a catheter be placed directly into the kidney or not? These decisions of treatment management for dying patients are dreadful and should if possible be made by the patient, with aware-

ness of her choices and prospects. In addition, Mrs. A. is very likely already suspicious that she is gravely ill, and we have no means of dealing with her fears without the ability to speak to her openly. Finally, the fears that the family expresses about the manner of informing her—"How can we tell our mother, 'You have cancer, it will kill you in weeks' "—are groundless: she must be told that she is very ill, but we would never advise telling her she has a period of x weeks to live—a statement that is never wise or medically sound—nor will we try to remove her hope.

The physician or other health care provider may be primarily motivated by the ethical principle of respect for patient autonomy, grounding a patient's right to know of his or her situation, choices, and likely fate. Connected with this may be the correct belief that any consent to treatment that the patient provides without having an opportunity to learn the reason for that treatment is legally invalid. To be properly informed, consent must be predicated on information about the nature and consequences of treatment, which must in turn be understood in the context of the patient's illness. A patient cannot validly consent to the passing of a tube into the kidney without being informed that her urinary tract is blocked, or of the reason for that blockage.

These reasons, so determinative for the physician, often carry no weight with the family. In Mrs. A.'s case, for example, the family pledged to sign anything we would like to free us of liability. Our response, that their willingness cannot affect either our moral or legal obligation, which vests in the patient directly, was similarly unpersuasive; nonetheless, it was a fact and had to be said.

The direct negative impact on the patient's care and comfort that results from her being left in the dark represents more in the way of common ground between family and health care provider. It is often quite clear that failure to reveal the truth causes a variety of unfortunate psychosocial results. As in all such cases, we highlighted for Mrs. A.'s family the strong possibility that she already suspects she is ill and dying of cancer but is unable to speak about this with them because all of us, in our concealment and evasions, had not given her "permission" to broach the topic. Mrs. A. is dying, but there are things worse than dying, for example, dying in silence when one needs to speak.

It is also important to emphasize to families that the patient may have "unfinished business" that he or she would like to complete. For example, after one of my earliest consultations of this nature, the patient in question chose to leave the hospital for several weeks to revisit his birthplace in Greece.

Finally, it is sometimes the case that the failure to discuss with the patient his or her diagnosis can directly result in inadequate or inappropriate medical care. Mrs. S., above, was denied adequate comfort measures because the institution of morphine might tip her off to her condition. In another case, the son and daughter-in-law of a patient insisted that she not receive chemotherapy for an advanced but treatable blood cancer so that she would be spared the knowledge of her disease and the side effects of treatment. In such cases, great injury is added to the insult of withholding the truth from a patient. Often, it is this prospect that serves as the trigger to mobilize the health care team to seek an ethical consultation.

### Offering Truth to the Uninformed Patient with Cancer

A patient's knowledge of diagnosis and prognosis is not all-or-nothing. It exists along a continuum, anchored at one end by the purely theoretical "absolute ignorance" and at the other by the unattainable "total enlightenment." Actual patients are to be found along this continuum at locations that vary in response to external factors (verbal information, nonverbal clues, etc.) as well as internal dynamics, such as denial.

The approach called here "offering truth" represents a brief dance between patient and health care provider, a pas de deux, that takes place within that continuum. When offering truth to the patient with cancer, rather than simply ascertaining that the patient is for the moment lucid, and then proceeding to explain all aspects of his or her condition and treatment, both the physician(s) and I attempt repeatedly to ascertain from the patient how much he or she wants to know. In dealing with families who insist that the patient remain uninformed, I explain this approach, a kind of compromise between the polar stances. I also explain that sometimes the results are surprising, as indeed happened with Mrs. A.

> In spite of all the explanations we provided to Mrs. A.'s family of the many reasons why it might be best to speak with her of her illness, they continued to resist. Mrs. A., the son insisted, would want all the decisions that arise to be made by the physicians, whom they all trusted, and the family itself.
>
> If their assessment of Mrs. A. is correct, I pointed out, we have no

problem. Dr. H. agrees with me that while Mrs. A. has a *right* to know, she does not have a *duty* to know. We would not force this information on her—indeed, we cannot. Patients who do not want to know will sometimes deny ever having been told, however forthrightly they have been spoken to. So Mrs. A. will be offered this information, not have it thrust on her—and if they are right about what she wants, and her personality, she will not wish to know.

Mrs. A. was awake and reasonably alert, although not altogether free of discomfort (nausea). She was told that she had had an infection that was now under control, but that she remains very ill, as she herself can tell from her weakness. Does she have any questions she wants to ask; does she want to talk? She did not. We repeated that she remains very ill and asked if she understands that—she did. Some patients, it was explained to her, want to know all about their disease—its name, prognosis, treatment choices, famous people who have had the disease, etc.—while others do not want to know so much, and some want to leave all of the decisions in the hands of their family and physicians. What would she like? What kind of patient is she? She whispered to her daughter that she wants to leave it alone for now.

That seemed to be her final word. We repeated to her that treatment choices would need to be made shortly. She was told that we would respect her desire, but that if she changed her mind we could talk at any time; and that, in any event, she must understand that we would stay by her and see to her comfort in all possible ways. She signified that she understood and said that we should deal with her children. Both Dr. H. and I understood this as explicitly authorizing her children to speak for her with respect to treatment decisions.

The above approach relies on one simple tactic: a patient will be offered the opportunity to learn the truth, at whatever level of detail that patient desires. The most important step in these attempts is to ask questions of the patient and then listen closely to the patient's responses. Since the discussion at hand concerns how much information the patient would like to receive, here, unlike most physician-patient interchanges, the important decisions will need to be made by the patient.

Initiating discussion is relatively easy if the patient is only recently conscious and responsive; it is more difficult if a conspiracy of silence has already taken effect. The conversation with the patient might be initiated by telling him or her that at this time the medical team has arrived at a fairly clear understanding of the situation and treatment options. New test results may be alluded to; this is a fairly safe statement, since new tests are always being done on all patients. These conversational gambits signal that a fresh start in communication can now be attempted. (At the same time it avoids the awkwardness of a patient's asking, "Why haven't you spoken to me before?")

The patient might then be told that, before we talk about our current understanding of the medical situation, it is important to hear from the patient himself or herself, so that we can confirm what he or she knows or clear up any misunderstanding that may have arisen. The patient sometimes, with more than a little logic, responds, "Why are you asking me what is wrong? You're the doctor, you tell me what's wrong." A variety of answers are possible. A patient might be told that we have found that things work better if we start with the patient's understanding of the illness; or that time might be saved if we know what the patient understands, and go from there; or that whenever you try to teach someone, you have to start with what they know. Different approaches may suggest themselves as more fitting to the particular patient in question. The important thing is to begin to generate a dynamic within which the patient is speaking and the physician responding, rather than vice versa. Only then can the pace of conversation and level of information be controlled by the patient. The structure of the discussion, as well as the content of what the physician says, must reinforce the message: We are now establishing a new opportunity to talk and question, but you as the patient will have to tell us how much you want to know about your illness.

The chief ethical principle underlying the idea that patients should be offered the truth is, of course, respect for the patient's personal autonomy. By holding the conversation, the patient is given the opportunity to express autonomy in its most robust, direct fashion: the clear expression of preference. Legal systems that value autonomy will similarly protect a physician who chooses to offer truth and to respect the patient's response to that offer; "a medical doctor need not make disclosure of risks when the patient requests that he not be so informed."[5] A patient's right to information vests in that patient, to exercise as he or she desires; so that a patient's right to information is respected no less when the patient chooses to be relatively uninformed as when full information is demanded.[6] This stance is entirely consistent with the recent adoption of the widely noted (and even more widely misconstrued) Patient Self-Determination Act.[7]

The major innovation this entails has been to involve institutions in the process of informing patients of their rights. However, the Patient Self-Determination Act has not changed state laws about informed consent to treatment in any way,[8] and as such the basic question here addressed—a physician's responsibility to inform patients of their diagnoses—remains entirely unaffected.

When offering truth, we are forced to recognize that patients' choices should be respected not because we or others agree with those choices (still less, respected *only* when we agree with those choices), but simply because those are the patient's choices. Indeed, the test of autonomy comes precisely when we personally disagree with the path the patient had chosen. If, for example, patient choice is respected only when the patient chooses the most effective treatment, when respecting those choices we would be respecting only effective therapeutics, not the person who has chosen them.

Many physicians hold to the ideal of an informed, alert, cooperative, and intelligent patient. But the point of offering truth—rather than inflicting it—is to allow the patient to choose his or her own path. As a practical matter, of course, it could scarcely be otherwise. A physician with fanatic devotion to informing patients can lecture, explain, even harangue, but cannot force the patient to attend to what the physician is saying, or think about it, or remember it.

Families need to confront the same point. Ambivalence and conflict are often observed among family members concerning whether the patient who has not been informed "really" knows (or suspects, etc.), and by offering the patient the opportunity to speak, this issue may be settled. More fundamentally, though, the concealing family—which is after all characterized by deep concern for the patient's well-being—will rarely (has never, in my experience to date) maintain that even if the patient demands to know the truth, the secret should still be kept. The family rather relies on the patient's failure to make this explicit demand as his or her tacit agreement to remain ignorant. Families can be helped to see that there may be many reasons for the patient's failure to demand the truth (including the fact that the patient may believe the lies that have been offered). If the patient wishes to remain in a state of relative ignorance, he or she will tell us that when asked; and if the patient states an explicit desire to be informed, families will find it hard to deny his or her right to have that desire respected.

Some families, naturally enough, suspect chicanery, that this approach is rigged to get the patient to ask for the truth. To them I respond that my experience proves otherwise: to my surprise and that of the physicians, some patients ask to leave this in the family's hands; to the surprise of families, some patients who seemed quietistic in fact strongly wish to be told the truth (which many of them had already suspected). We cannot know what the patient wants until we ask, I tell them, and we all want to do what the patient wants.

Having held the discussion, it is important to move on to its resolution as soon as possible.

> I met with Mrs. S.'s children, together with a nurse, medical resident, and medical student, for about an hour and a half; the treating oncologist also made a brief appearance. The discussion featured a lengthy and eloquent exposition by the resident of why Mrs. S. needs to be spoken to, and a passionate and equally eloquent appeal by one son to respect the different culture from which they come. Finally, I introduced the idea that we offer her the truth, and then follow her lead. This was agreed to by the family, and I left.

The medical student thanked me some days later and told me the rest of the story. The tension that had existed between health care team and family had largely dissipated; as the student put it, "People were able to look each other in the eye again." Mrs. S. was lucid but fatigued that evening; for that reason, and probably because they had already spent so much time talking at our meeting, the family delayed the agreed-on discussion. Unexpectedly, Mrs. S. did not survive the night.

## Conclusion

The problem of the uninformed patient with cancer can be described in many different ways, for example, as faulty physician-patient communication; as an obstacle to good medical care; as a cause of stress among hospital staff; and as a failure to respect patient autonomy. A dimension at least as important as these, but rarely acknowledged, is the clash it may represent between diverse cultures and their basic moral commitments.

The approach presented above reflects an effort to maintain accepted standards of the physician-patient relationship while respecting the cultural background and requirements of families. This form of respect involves reasonable accommodation to these cultural expectations but should not be confused with uncritical acquiescence. The critical question is, perhaps, this: How should we react to a family that refuses to allow the patient an offering of truth, that maintains that discussion itself to be contrary to cultural norms? Under those circumstances, I believe the offering must be made notwithstanding family demands. My reasons have as much to do with my beliefs about the nature of ethnic and religious moral norms themselves as with the view that in cases of conflict, our public morality (as concretized in law) should prevail.

First, I believe that members of a cultural community are as prone to mistaking what their own norms require of them as we within the broader culture are to mistaking our own moral obligations. The norm of protecting the patient clearly requires rather than prohibits disclosure in some cases, including some described above, to prevent physical or psychological damage or to enable some final task to be consummated. All of the factors that we recognize sometimes to derange our own moral judgments—inertia, ill-grounded prejudices and generalizations, lack of the courage to confront unpleasant situations, and many more—may operate as powerfully in deranging the views of those from another culture. Their initial sense of what ethics require may, that is, be mistaken, from the point of view of their own norms as well as those of modern, Western, secular culture.

Second, even if a family's judgment of what their culture requires is accurate, we must not presume that a patient like Mrs. A. will choose, in extremis, to abide by her own cultural norms. Like any immigrant, she may have adopted the norms of broad society, or, acculturated to some lesser degree, she may act according to some hybrid set of values. Concretely, the offering of truth is about her diagnosis; symbolically, it is a process that allows her to declare her own preference regarding which norms shall be respected and how.

A last word is in order about the view implicit in this approach regarding the nature of a bioethical consultation. As these cases illustrate, patients, families, and health care professionals come to a meeting from different moral worlds, as well as different backgrounds and biographies; and these worlds involve not simply rights and privileges, but duties as well. A successful consultation attempts to clarify on behalf of the different parties their own moral principles and associated moral commitments. It needs to proceed from the premise that all present ultimately share a common goal: the well-being of the patient.

## Notes

I am grateful to Eugene V. Bareza, MD, CM, and to Charles Weijer, MD, for valuable advice in the preparation of the manuscript. All errors are my own.

1 Oken, D. What to tell cancer patients: a study of medical attitudes. *JAMA*. 1961;175:1120–1128.

2 Novack, D.H., Plumer, R., Smith, R.L., Ochitil, H., Morrow, G.R., Bennett, J.M. Changes in physicians' attitudes toward telling the cancer patient. *JAMA*. 1979;241:897–900.

3 Welts, E.P. The Greek family. In: McGoldrick, M.M., Pearce, J.K., Giordano, J. *Ethnicity and Family Therapy*. New York: Guilford Press: 1982:269–288.

4 Dalla-Vorgia, P., Katsouyanni, K., Garanis, T.N., et al. Attitudes of a Mediterranean population to the truth-telling issue. *J Med Ethics*. 1992;18:67–74.

5 *Cobbs v Grant*. 502 P2d 1 (Cal 1972) (a similar provision for a patient's right to waive being informed was established by the Supreme Court of Canada in *Reibl v. Hughes* 2SCR 880 [1980]).

6 Freedman, B. The validity of ignorant consent to medical research. *IRB Rev Hum Subjects Res*. 1982;4(2):1–5.

7 The Patient Self Determination Act, sections 4206 and 4751 of the Omnibus Reconciliation Act of 1990, Pub L 101–508.

8 McCloskey, E. Between isolation and intrusion: the Patient Self Determination Act. *Law Med Health Care*. 1991;19:80–82.

## What the Doctor Said
Raymond Carver

He said it doesn't look good
he said it looks bad in fact real bad
he said I counted thirty-two of them on one lung before
I quit counting them
I said I'm glad I wouldn't want to know
about any more being there than that
he said are you a religious man do you kneel down
in forest groves and let yourself ask for help
when you come to a waterfall
mist blowing against your face and arms
do you stop and ask for understanding at those moments
I said not yet but I intend to start today
he said I'm real sorry he said
I wish I had some other kind of news to give you
I said Amen and he said something else
I didn't catch and not knowing what else to do
and not wanting him to have to repeat it
and me to have to fully digest it
I just looked at him
for a minute and he looked back it was then
I jumped up and shook hands with this man who'd just given me
something no one else on earth had ever given me
I may even have thanked him habit being so strong

# PART IV

**The End of Life**

## A Man in His Life
Yehuda Amichai

A man doesn't have time in his life
to have time for everything.
He doesn't have seasons enough to have
a season for every purpose. Ecclesiastes
was wrong about that.

A man needs to love and to hate at the same moment,
to laugh and cry with the same eyes,
with the same hands to throw stones and to gather them,
to make love in war and war in love.

And to hate and forgive and remember and forget,
to arrange and confuse, to eat and to digest
what history
takes years and years to do.

A man doesn't have time.
When he loses he seeks, when he finds
he forgets, when he forgets he loves, when he loves
he begins to forget.

Yehuda Amichai, "A Man in His Life," from *The Selected Poetry of Yehuda Amichai*, trans.
Chana Bloch and Stephan Mitchell, © 1986 by Yehuda Amichai. Reprinted by permission of
University of California Press.

And his soul is seasoned, his soul
is very professional.
Only his body remains forever
an amateur. It tries and it misses,
gets muddled, doesn't learn a thing,
drunk and blind in its pleasures
and its pains.

He will die as figs die in autumn,
Shriveled and full of himself and sweet,
the leaves growing dry on the ground,
the bare branches pointing to the place
where there's time for everything.

## End-of-Life Ethics: Some
## Common Definitions
Larry R. Churchill and
Nancy M. P. King

*Euthanasia.* The deliberate taking of a life by active means, such as a lethal injection. Acts of euthanasia can be voluntary, meaning with patient consent, or nonvoluntary, denoting the absence of consent, as when the patient is unconscious or otherwise unable to make a request. Voluntary euthanasia is legally permitted in the Netherlands when performed by physicians under carefully circumscribed conditions. Dutch physicians receive roughly 5,000 patient requests for euthanasia annually, with "pain" and "deterioration" being the most frequently cited reasons. While Dutch laws now protect physicians from criminal prosecution, the population has been openly tolerant of such practices since the mid-1970s. Euthanasia, whether voluntary or nonvoluntary, is illegal in the United States and not condoned in any code of medical ethics.

*Physician-assisted suicide (PAS).* The act of assisting a patient in taking his/her own life, for example, by providing a prescription and information on the lethal dose of a medication. PAS can exist along a broad continuum of actions. In some situations, the assistance of physicians can be small, for example, responding to a request for information. In other situations, the assistance can be so large as to be practically indistinguishable from active killing of patients, as in the actions of Dr. Jack Kevorkian, who hooked patients up to all the necessary machinery for delivering a lethal intervention, leaving only the pushing of a button in the patient's hands. PAS, defined as providing a lethal prescription, is currently legal in Oregon when specific guidelines are followed, including a time delay and second-opinion requirement to safeguard against abuse. Bills to legalize PAS failed by narrow margins in both California and Washington in the 1990s. American physicians are divided on both the morality of PAS and the desirability of legalization, mirroring the division of opinion in the general public.

*Allowing to die through withdrawal of treatment/palliation that hastens time of death.* While active euthanasia and PAS are rare occurrences, patients who die in hospitals, nursing homes, or hospices almost always have the timing of their deaths managed or orchestrated in a variety of ways. Most important among these is removing—or not starting—life-sustaining treatments that are no longer considered beneficial, that the patient does not want, or that present greater burdens than benefits. A great many deaths in institutions are also accompanied by provision of medications to alleviate pain and suffering that may hasten death. This has been an accepted practice since the beginning of Western medicine; relief of suffering at the end of life is considered one of medicine's most important responsibilities. Hastening the time of death for a terminally ill person through appropriate pain control is not considered euthanasia, and is morally and legally accepted virtually universally. The U.S. Supreme Court, in *Washington v. Glucksberg* (1997), put it this way: "A person facing a painful death has no legal barriers to obtaining medication, from qualified physicians, even to the point of causing unconsciousness and hastening death."

*Brain death.* More properly termed "death by neurological criteria," brain death is defined as death of the whole brain, including the brain stem. Brain death is legally death in the United States, by statute, although in at least one state it is statutorily permissible to raise religious objections to brain death criteria. Brain death was first introduced to the medical profession in 1968, as the product of a Harvard Medical School committee establishing criteria and tests for "irreversible coma." Variations on the tests described therein, including serial EEGs separated by a prescribed interval, are still in general use. The medical/moral reasons for developing this alternative to traditional determinations of death by heart-lung criteria were that the technological ability to preserve heart and lung function artificially made it impossible to determine death without causing it, and that loss of function of the whole brain and brain stem resulted in permanent cessation of all meaningful neurological activity and irreversible deterioration of integrative physiological functioning. The policy reason was to facilitate cadaveric organ donation, since death by neurological criteria is declared before interventions supporting heart and lung function are removed. Brain death is currently recognized and accepted, to varying degrees, throughout the world. Nonetheless, popular and professional confusion about the concept persists (newspaper headlines like "Brain-dead woman kept alive to give birth" are still common), demonstrating that death is as much a cultural as a scientific concept. Moreover, there is increasing evidence that neurological death may be a more complex process than was originally appreciated. Despite these caveats, death by neurological criteria seems well established, both scientifically and as a matter of policy. Debates about the appropriateness of extending the definition of death to higher-brain (cortical) death continue.

*Persistent vegetative state (pvs).* A condition of irreversible loss of cortical activity without loss of autonomic (brain stem) functioning. Patients in pvs lack consciousness, self-awareness, and awareness of their surroundings, but retain some reflexes (such as certain reactions to light and pain) and have heart and lung function. Some patients in pvs can be kept alive for many years with artificial nutrition and hydration. pvs is not coma; patients in pvs have sleep-wake cycles, and may therefore appear to have minimal cortical function. Although patients can awaken from coma, even after many years, pvs when properly diagnosed is considered irreversible. Karen Ann Quinlan was the first patient widely known to be in pvs. After her family won the legal right to have her removed from respiratory support in 1976, on the grounds that she would have chosen death instead of being burdened with an intervention that could keep her alive but not restore her to consciousness, she was successfully weaned from respiratory support and lived on in pvs for years. pvs has remained controversial, even reaching the U.S. Supreme Court in 1990 in the case of Nancy Cruzan. In almost all states, patients who have written living wills or named health care agents to act for them may through these advance directives refuse artificial nutrition and hydration if in pvs. However, in some states, women's advance directives refusing treatment in pvs are invalidated by statute during pregnancy, in order to preserve the fetal environment. Profound disagreements about the meaning and value of life in pvs have resulted in many public controversies, such as the case of Theresa Schiavo in Florida.

# Informed Demand for
# "Non-Beneficial" Medical Treatment
Steven H. Miles

An 85-year-old woman was taken from a nursing home to Hennepin County Medical Center on January 1, 1990, for emergency treatment of dyspnea from chronic bronchiectasis. The patient, Mrs. Helga Wanglie, required emergency intubation and was placed on a respirator. She occasionally acknowledged discomfort and recognized her family but could not communicate clearly. In May, after attempts to wean her from the respirator failed, she was discharged to a chronic care hospital. One week later, her heart stopped during a weaning attempt; she was resuscitated and taken to another hospital for intensive care. She remained unconscious, and a physician suggested that it would be appropriate to consider withdrawing life support. In response, the family transferred her back to the medical center on May 31. Two weeks later, physicians concluded that she was in a persistent vegetative state as a result of severe anoxic encephalopathy. She was maintained on a respirator, with repeated courses of antibiotics, frequent airway suctioning, tube feedings, an air flotation bed, and biochemical monitoring.

In June and July of 1990, physicians suggested that life-sustaining treatment be withdrawn since it was not benefiting the patient. Her husband, daughter, and son insisted on continued treatment. They stated their view that physicians should not play God, that the patient would not be better off dead, that removing life support showed moral decay in our civilization, and that a miracle could occur. Her husband told a physician that his wife had never stated her preferences concerning life-sustaining treatment. He believed that the cardiac arrest would not have occurred if she

Steven Miles, "Informed Demand for 'Non-Beneficial' Medical Treatment," from *New England Journal of Medicine*, vol. 325, 512–515. © 1991 by the Massachusetts Medical Society. Reprinted by permission of the publisher.

had not been transferred from Hennepin County Medical Center in May. The family reluctantly accepted a do-not-resuscitate order based on the improbability of Mrs. Wanglie's surviving a cardiac arrest. In June, an ethics committee consultant recommended continued counseling for the family. The family declined counseling, including the counsel of their own pastor, and in late July asked that the respirator not be discussed again. In August, nurses expressed their consensus that continued life support did not seem appropriate, and I, as the newly appointed ethics consultant, counseled them.

In October 1990, a new attending physician consulted with specialists and confirmed the permanence of the patient's cerebral and pulmonary conditions. He concluded that she was at the end of her life and that the respirator was "non-beneficial," in that it could not heal her lungs, palliate her suffering, or enable this unconscious and permanently respirator-dependent woman to experience the benefit of the life afforded by respirator support. Because the respirator could prolong life, it was not character-ized as "futile."[1] In November, the physician, with my concurrence, told the family that he was not willing to continue to prescribe the respirator. The husband, an attorney, rejected proposals to transfer the patient to another facility or to seek a court order mandating this unusual treatment. The hospital told the family that it would ask a court to decide whether members of its staff were obliged to continue treatment. A second con-ference two weeks later, after the family had hired an attorney, confirmed these positions, and the husband asserted that the patient had consistently said she wanted respirator support for such a condition.

In December, the medical director and hospital administrator asked the Hennepin County Board of Commissioners (the medical center's board of directors) to allow the hospital to go to court to resolve the dispute. In January, the county board gave permission by a 4-to-3 vote. Neither the hospital nor the county had a financial interest in terminating treat-ment. Medicare largely financed the $200,000 for the first hospitalization at Hennepin County; a private insurer would pay the $500,000 bill for the second. From February through May of 1991, the family and its at-torney unsuccessfully searched for another health care facility that would admit Mrs. Wanglie. Facilities with empty beds cited her poor potential for rehabilitation.

The hospital chose a two-step legal procedure, first asking for the ap-pointment of an independent conservator to decide whether the respirator was beneficial to the patient and, second, if the conservator found it was not, for a second hearing on whether it was obliged to provide the respirator. The husband cross-filed, requesting to be appointed conservator. After a hearing in late May, the trial court on July 1, 1991, appointed the husband, as best able to represent the patient's interests. It noted that no request to stop treatment had been made and declined to speculate on the legality of such an order.[2] The hospital said that it would continue to provide the respirator in the light of continuing uncertainty about its legal obligation to provide it. Three days later, despite aggressive care, the patient died of multisystem organ failure resulting from septicemia. The family declined an autopsy and stated that the patient had received excellent care.

### Discussion

This sad story illustrates the problem of what to do when a family demands medical treatment that the attending physician concludes cannot benefit the patient. Only 600 elderly people are treated with respirators for more than six months in the United States each year.[3] Presumably, most of these people are actually or potentially conscious. It is common practice to discontinue the use of a respirator before death when it can no longer benefit a patient.[4,5]

We do not know Mrs. Wanglie's treatment preferences. A large majority of elderly people prefer not to receive prolonged respirator support for irreversible unconsciousness.[6] Studies show that an older person's designated family proxy overestimates that person's preference for life-sustaining treatment in a hypothetical coma.[7-9] The implications of this research for clinical decision making have not been cogently analyzed.

A patient's request for a treatment does not necessarily oblige a provider or the health care system. Patients may not demand that physicians injure them (for example, by mutilation), or provide plausible but inappropriate therapies (for example, amphetamines for weight reduction), or therapies that have no value (such as laetrile for cancer). Physicians are not obliged to violate their personal moral views on medical care so long as patients' rights are served. Minnesota's Living Will law says that physicians are "legally bound to act consistently within [the patient's] wishes within limits of reasonable medical practice" in acting on requests and refusals of treatment.[10] Minnesota's Bill of Patients' Rights says that patients "have the right to appropriate medical . . . care based on individual needs . . . [which is] limited where the service is not reimbursable."[11] Mrs. Wanglie also had aortic insufficiency. Had this condition worsened, a surgeon's refusal to perform a life-prolonging valve replacement as medically inappropriate would hardly occasion public controversy. As the Minneapolis *Star Tribune* said in an editorial on the eve of the trial,

> The hospital's plea is born of realism, not hubris. . . . It advances the claim that physicians should not be slaves to technology—any more than patients should be its prisoners. They should be free to deliver, and act on, an honest and time-honored message: "Sorry, there's nothing more we can do."[12]

Disputes between physicians and patients about treatment plans are often handled by transferring patients to the care of other providers. In this case, every provider contacted by the hospital or the family refused to treat this patient with a respirator. These refusals occurred before and after this case became a matter of public controversy and despite the availability of third-party reimbursement. We believe they represent a medical consensus that respirator support is inappropriate in such a case.

The handling of this case is compatible with current practices regarding informed consent, respect for patients' autonomy, and the right to health care. Doctors should inform patients of all medically reasonable treatments, even those available from other providers. Patients can refuse any prescribed treatment or choose among any medical alternatives that physicians are willing to prescribe. Respect for autonomy does not empower patients to oblige physicians to prescribe treatments in ways that are fruitless or inappropriate. Previous "right to die" cases address the different situation of a patient's right to choose to be free of a prescribed therapy. This case is more about the nature of the patient's entitlement to treatment than about the patient's choice in using that entitlement.

The proposal that this family's preference for this unusual and costly treatment, which is commonly regarded as inappropriate, establishes a right to such treatment is ironic, given that preference does not create a right to other needed, efficacious, and widely desired treatments in the United States. We could not afford a universal health care system based on patients' demands. Such a system would irrationally allocate health care to socially powerful people with strong preferences for immediate treatment to the disadvantage of those with less power or less immediate needs.

After the conclusion was reached that the respirator was not benefiting the patient, the decision to seek a review of the duty to provide it was based on an ethic of "stewardship." Even though the insurer played no part in this case, physicians' discretion to prescribe requires responsible handling of requests for inappropriate treatment. Physicians exercise this stewardship by counseling against or denying such treatment or by submitting such requests to external review. This stewardship is not aimed at protecting the assets of insurance companies but rests on fairness to people who have pooled their resources to insure their collective access to appropriate health care. Several citizens complained to Hennepin County Medical Center that Mrs. Wanglie was receiving expensive treatment paid for by people who had not consented to underwrite a level of medical care whose appropriateness was defined by family demands.

Procedures for addressing this kind of dispute are at an early stage of development. Though the American Medical Association[13] and the Society of Critical Care Medicine[14] also support some decisions to withhold requested treatment, the medical center's reasoning most closely follows the guidelines of the American Thoracic Society.[15] The statements of these professional organizations do not clarify when or how a physician may legally withdraw or withhold demanded life-sustaining treatments. The request for a conservator to review the medical conclusion before considering the medical obligation was often misconstrued as implying that the husband was incompetent or ill motivated. The medical center intended to emphasize the desirability of an independent review of its medical conclusion before its obligation to provide the respirator was reviewed by the court. I believe that the grieving husband was simply mistaken about whether the respirator was benefiting his wife. A direct request to remove the respirator seems to center procedural oversight on the soundness of the medical decision making rather than on the nature of the patient's need. Clearly, the gravity of these decisions merits openness, due process, and meticulous accountability. The relative merits of various procedures need further study.

Ultimately, procedures for addressing requests for futile, marginally effective, or inappropriate therapies require a statutory framework, case law, professional standards, a social consensus, and the exercise of professional responsibility. Appropriate ends for medicine are defined by public and professional consensus. Laws can, and do, say that patients may choose only among medically appropriate options, but legislatures are ill suited to define medical appropriateness. Similarly, health facility policies on this issue will be difficult to design and will focus on due process rather than on specific clinical situations. Public or private payers will ration according to cost and overall efficacy, a rationing that will become more onerous as therapies are misapplied in individual cases. I believe there is a social consensus that intensive care for a person as "overmastered" by disease as this woman was is inappropriate.

Each case must be evaluated individually. In this case, the husband's request seemed entirely inconsistent with what medical care could do for his wife, the standards of the community, and his fair share of resources that many people pooled for their collective medical care. This case is about limits to what can be achieved at the end of life.

## Notes

1   Tomlinson, T., Brody, H. Futility and the ethics of resuscitation. JAMA 1990; 264:1276–80.
2   In re Helga Wanglie, Fourth Judicial District (Dist. Ct., Probate Ct. Div.) PX-91-283. Minnesota, Hennepin County.
3   Office of Technology Assessment Task Force. Life-sustaining technologies and the elderly. Washington, D.C.: Government Printing Office, 1987.
4   Smedira, N.G., Evans, B.H., Grais, L.S., et al. Withholding and withdrawal of life support from the critically ill. N Engl J Med 1990; 322:309–15.
5   Lantos, J.D., Singer, P.A., Walker, R.M., et al. The illusion of futility in clinical practice. Am J Med 1989; 87-81-4.
6   Emanuel, L.L., Barry, M.J., Stoeckle, J.D., Ettelson, L.M., Emanuel, E.J. Advance directives for medical care—a case for greater use. N Engl J Med 1991; 324: 889–95.
7   Zweibel, N.R., Cassel, C.K. Treatment choices at the end of life: a comparison of decisions by older patients and their physician-selected proxies. Gerontologist 1989; 29:615–21.
8   Tomlinson, T., Howe, K., Notman, M., Rossmiller, D. An empirical study of proxy consent for elderly persons. Gerontologist 1990; 30:54–64.
9   Danis, M., Southerland, L.I., Garrett, J.M., et al. A prospective study of advance directives for life-sustaining care. N Engl J Med 1991; 324:882–8.
10  Minnesota Statutes. Adult Health Care Decisions Act. 145b.04.
11  Minnesota Statutes. Patients and residents of health care facilities; Bill of rights. 144.651: Subd. 6.
12  Helga Wanglie's life. Minneapolis Star Tribune. May 26, 1991:18A.
13  Council on Ethical and Judicial Affairs, American Medical Association. Guidelines for the appropriate use of do-not-resuscitate orders. JAMA 1991; 265: 1868–71.
14  Task Force on Ethics of the Society of Critical Care Medicine. Consensus report on the ethics of foregoing life-sustaining treatments in the critically ill. Crit Care Med 1990; 18:1435–9.
15  American Thoracic Society. Withholding and withdrawing life-sustaining therapy. Am Rev Respir Dis 1992.

# The Case of Helga Wanglie:
## A New Kind of "Right to Die" Case
Marcia Angell

Helga Wanglie, an 86-year-old Minneapolis woman, died of sepsis on July 4 after being in a persistent vegetative state for over a year. She was the focus of an extremely important controversy over the right to die that culminated in a court decision just three days before her death.[1] The controversy pitted her husband and children, who wanted her life maintained on a respirator, against doctors at the Hennepin County Medical Center, who wanted her removed from the respirator because they regarded the treatment as inappropriate. The judge decided in favor of Mr. Wanglie, and Helga Wanglie died still supported by the respirator.

The Wanglie case differed in a crucial way from earlier right-to-die cases, beginning with the case of Karen Quinlan 16 years ago. In the earlier cases, the families wished to withhold life-sustaining treatment and the institutions had misgivings. Here it was the reverse; the family wanted to continue life-sustaining treatment, not to stop it, and the institution argued for the right to die. Mr. Wanglie believed that life should be maintained as long as possible, no matter what the circumstances, and he asserted that his wife shared this belief.

In one sense, the court's opinion in the Wanglie case would seem to be at odds with most of the earlier opinions in that it resulted in continued treatment of a patient in a persistent vegetative state. In another sense, however, the opinion was quite consistent, because it affirmed the right of the family to make decisions about life-sustaining treatment when the patient was no longer able to do so. By granting guardianship of

Marcia Angell, "The Case of Helga Wanglie: A New Kind of 'Right to Die' Case," from *New England Journal of Medicine*, vol. 325, 511–512. © 1991 by the Massachusetts Medical Society. Reprinted by permission of the publisher. All rights reserved.

Mrs. Wanglie to her husband, the judge indicated that the most important consideration was who made the decision, not what the decision was. I believe that this was wise; any other decision by the court would have been inimical to patient autonomy and would have undermined the consensus on the right to die that has been carefully crafted since the Quinlan case.

What are the elements of that consensus and how should they be applied to the Wanglie case and others like it? There is general agreement that competent adults may refuse any recommended medical care. This right, based on principles of self-determination, has repeatedly been buttressed by the courts. When patients are no longer mentally competent, families are to act in accordance with what the patient would wish (a principle known as substituted judgment).[2-4] Disputes have arisen, however, when the patient had not, while competent, clearly expressed his or her preferences. This was the situation in the Wanglie case, as it was thought to be in the Cruzan case.[5]

To avoid these disputes, there is a growing movement to encourage all adults to prepare a document that would provide guidance, if necessary, for their families and doctors.[6] Such documents include living wills, durable powers of attorney, and other instruments that have been specially devised for the purpose. Congress recently mandated that as of December 1991, all health care facilities must provide an opportunity for patients to prepare such a document on admission.

We are still left with the problem of deciding for those who have nevertheless provided no guidance, including those who were unable to do so, such as children or profoundly retarded adults. In these cases as well, families usually make decisions on behalf of the patient, but since the patient's wishes are unknown, the consensus holds that the family's decision must be consistent with the patient's best interests.[2-4] A decision consistent with best interests is usually defined as a choice that reasonable adults might make if faced with the problem. This is a vague but useful standard that, by definition, restricts the range of permissible decisions. It can, however, allow for more than one possible choice. For example, the decision to withdraw the respirator from Karen Quinlan was thought by the New Jersey Supreme Court to be consistent with her best interests, but her father was given the latitude to decide either way.[7]

The well-publicized legal disputes involving the right to die—such as the Quinlan case, the Brophy case in Massachusetts,[8] and the Cruzan case in Missouri—have reached the courts either because the institution believed it improper to withhold life-sustaining treatment at the family's request or because the institution wanted legal immunity before doing so. Until the Wanglie case, there was only one well-publicized case of the reverse situation—that is, of a family wishing to persist in treatment over the objections of the institution. This was the poignant case of Baby L, described last year in the *Journal*.[9] The case involved a two-year-old child, profoundly retarded and completely immobile, who required repeated cardiopulmonary resuscitation for survival. Baby L's mother insisted that this be done as often as necessary, despite the fact that there was no hope of recovery. Representatives of the hospital challenged her decision in court on the grounds that the continued treatment caused great suffering to the child and thus violated its best interests. Before the court reached a decision, however, the mother transferred the child to a hospital that agreed to continue the treatment, and the case became legally moot.

Unlike the case of Baby L, the Wanglie case did not involve a course that would cause the patient great suffering. Because she was in a persistent vegetative state, Mrs. Wanglie was incapable of suffering. Therefore, a compelling case could not be made that her best interests were being violated by continued use of the respirator. Instead, representatives of the institution invoked Mrs. Wanglie's best interests to make a weaker case: that the use of the respirator failed to serve Mrs. Wanglie's best interests and should therefore not be continued. It was suggested that a victory for Mr. Wanglie would mean that patients or their families could demand whatever treatment they wished, regardless of its efficacy. Many commentators also emphasized the enormous expense of maintaining a patient on life support when those resources are needed to care for people who would clearly benefit. In the previous essay, Steven H. Miles, MD, the ethics committee consultant at the Hennepin County Medical Center who was the petitioner in the Wanglie case, presents the arguments of the institution.[10] They are strong arguments that deserve to be examined, but I believe that they are on balance not persuasive.

It is generally agreed, as Miles points out, that patients or their surrogates do not have the right to demand any medical treatment they choose.[11,12] For example, a patient cannot insist that his doctor give him penicillin for a head cold. Patients' rights on this score are limited to refusing treatment or to choosing among effective ones. In the case of Helga Wanglie, the institution saw the respirator as "non-beneficial" because it would not restore her to consciousness. In the family's view, however, merely maintaining life was a worthy goal, and the respirator was not only effective toward that end, but essential.

Public opinion polls indicate that most people would not want their lives maintained in a persistent vegetative state. Many consider life in this state to be an indignity, and care givers often find caring for such patients demoralizing. It is important, however, to acknowledge that not everyone agrees with this view and it is a highly personal issue. For the decision to rest with the family is the most sensitive and workable approach, and it is the generally accepted one. Furthermore, a system in which life-sustaining treatment is discontinued over the objections of those who love the patient, on a case-by-case basis, would be callous. It can be argued on medical grounds that the definition of brain death should be legally extended to include a persistent vegetative state, but unless that is done universally we have no principled basis on which to override a family's decision in this kind of case. It is dismaying, of course, that resources are spent sustaining the lives of patients who will never be sentient, but we as a society would be on the slipperiest of slopes if we permitted ourselves to withdraw life support from a patient simply because it would save money.

Since the Quinlan case it has gradually been accepted that the particular decision is less important than a clear understanding of who should make it, and the Wanglie case underscores this approach. When self-determination is impossible or an unambiguous proxy decision is unavailable, the consensus is that the family should make the decision. To be meaningful, this approach requires that we be willing to accept decisions with which we disagree. Only if a decision appears to violate the best interests of a patient who left no guidance or could provide none, as in the case of Baby L, should it be challenged by the institution. Thus, the sources of decisions about refusing medical treatment are, in order of precedence, the patient, the patient's prior directives or designated proxy, and the patient's family. Decisions from each of these sources should reflect the following standards, respectively: immediate self-determination, self-determination exercised earlier, and the best interests of the patient. Institutions lie outside this hierarchy of decision making and should intervene by going to court only if they believe a decision violates these standards. Although I am sympathetic with the view of the doctors at the Hennepin County Medical Center, I agree with the court that they were wrong to try to impose it on the Wanglie family.

## Notes

1   In re Helga Wanglie, Fourth Judicial District (Dist. Ct., Probate Ct. Div.) PX-91-283. Minnesota, Hennepin County.

2   Society for the Right to Die. The physician and the hopelessly ill patient: legal, medical and ethical guidelines. New York: Society for the Right to Die, 1985.

3   Guidelines on the termination of life-sustaining treatment and the care of the dying: a report by the Hastings Center. Briarcliff Manor, N.Y.: Hastings Center, 1987.

4   President's Commission for the Study of Ethical Problems in Medicine and Biomedical and Behavioral Research. Deciding to forego life-sustaining treatment: a report on the ethical, medical, and legal issues in treatment decisions. Washington, D.C.: Government Printing Office, 1983.

5   Cruzan v. Harmon, 760 S.W.2d 408 (1988).

6   Annas, G.J. The health care proxy and the living will. N Engl J Med 1991; 324:1210-3.

7   In re Quinlan, 70 NJ 10, 355 A.2d 647 (1976).

8   Brophy v. New England Sinai Hospital, Inc. (Mass. Probate County Ct., Oct. 21, Nov. 29, 1985) 85E0009-G1.

9   Paris, J.J., Crone, R.K., Reardon F. Physicians' refusal of requested treatment: the case of Baby L. N Engl J Med 1990; 322:1012-5.

10  Miles, S.H. Informed demand for "non-beneficial" medical treatment. N Engl J Med 1991; 325:512-5.

11  Brett, A.S., McCullough, L.B. When patients request specific interventions: defining the limits of the physician's obligation. N Engl J Med 1986; 315:1347-51.

12  Blackhall, L.J. Must we always use CPR? N Engl J Med 1987; 317:1281-5.

## Disconnecting a Ventilator at the Request of a Patient Who Knows He Will Then Die: The Doctor's Anguish
Miles J. Edwards and Susan W. Tolle

Recently we assisted in withdrawing life support from a patient who had repeatedly asked to have his ventilator disconnected, even after being informed that he would then die. We found little in the medical literature to guide us, especially at the feeling level, so we are sharing our experience with the hope that others will find our emotional responses, reasoning, and procedures useful.

### The Case

Mr. Larson was a 67-year-old, obese white man. At 23 years of age he developed poliomyelitis and "spent six weeks in an iron lung." His neurologic recovery was virtually complete, and he resumed a reasonably normal life.

In November 1990, he noted the onset of rapidly progressive dyspnea and weakness in his extremities. A month later, he was hospitalized. He was endotracheally intubated and then underwent a tracheostomy to provide continuous mechanical ventilation. Numerous attempts to wean the patient from the ventilator always failed within one to two minutes. He was alert and frustrated by his ventilator dependence and demonstrated some symptoms of situational depression. After careful pulmonologic and neurologic evaluation, his condition was attributed to "post-polio syndrome."

When the patient asked if he would ever be able to live without the

Miles J. Edwards and Susan W. Tolle, "Disconnecting a Ventilator at the Request of a Patient Who Knows He Will Then Die: The Doctor's Anguish," in *Annals of Internal Medicine*, vol. 117, 254–256. © 1992 by Miles J. Edwards, Susan W. Tolle, and *Annals of Internal Medicine*. Reprinted by permission of the publisher and the authors.

ventilator, pulmonary and neurology consultants told him that he would always be ventilator-dependent. One consultant felt that he might improve enough to be taken off the ventilator during the day but that he would probably continue to need it at night. All consultants concurred that he would never become totally ventilator-independent. The patient listened and, after thinking it over, asked to have ventilatory support discontinued. He stated that he realized he would die without such support.

A psychiatrist evaluated the patient and agreed that he was somewhat depressed, although not severely enough to affect his decision-making capacity. After some initial reservations, the patient's family (one grown daughter and two grown sons) showed strong support for his decision. The patient consistently made it clear that living on continuous mechanical ventilation, with the consequent inability to speak, rendered the quality of his life unacceptable. He continued to express his wish to discontinue ventilation over a two-week period and asked to be heavily sedated in the process. Because of his unwavering request, we were called in as ethics consultants.

### Ensuring That Ventilator Withdrawal Is Right for the Patient

We believe that after careful consideration in selected cases, withdrawal of the ventilator from an awake patient, allowing a natural death to occur, is the right thing to do. We object to the term "passive euthanasia"; it is not killing the patient. It is instead stepping aside and allowing the disease to take its natural course when that course is the consistent choice of a competent patient. The question then is whether that choice is ethically supportable in a particular patient. What do we need to consider before making this decision? And if we do decide to disconnect the ventilator, how can that be done with compassion to minimize or eliminate the patient's suffering?

We accept the ethical and legal principles that patients have the right to refuse medical treatment, even when they may die as a result. However, we have an obligation to verify that the refusal of life-sustaining treatment is the durable request of a mentally competent, well-informed patient. In Mr. Larson's case, we needed more information before we could respond to his request. We identify seven actions that must be addressed before such a request should be acted on.

1. Clarify the prognosis.
2. Be assured of the patient's decision-making capacity (and of the ab-

sence of a medically significant depression that might temporarily affect his or her judgment).

3. Assure durability of the patient's wish.
4. Identify any coercive influences, either personal or financial.
5. Explore concurrence of all family members.
6. Explore concurrence of all members of the health care team.
7. Consider legal mandates.

During the one week of our consultation, we talked repeatedly to the patient, separately to all three children, and also to some close friends of the family. One son appeared to have some misgivings, but they really represented, as further inquiry revealed, his great unhappiness about his father's condition. After coming to terms with those feelings, he agreed with his father's decision. We continued to explore the attitudes of all family members. From an ethical perspective, the patient's wishes should be respected, and unanimous agreement from the family is not necessarily required. However, we did obtain unanimous agreement from the family in support of our patient's decision.

We concluded that for Mr. Larson, withdrawal of the ventilator was both legally and ethically supportable, recognizing the right of competent, informed adults to refuse medical treatment. Then came the particularly difficult question: How could this be done with compassion and with a minimum of suffering?

### Discontinuing Mechanical Ventilation in a Conscious Patient

#### The Patient's Right to Sedation

Discontinuing mechanical ventilation is a uniquely difficult process for the patient, the family, the physician, and other members of the health care team. Regardless of how strongly the patient may wish to have this done, the sudden feeling of suffocation that results leads to a visceral panic. This sensation constitutes the greatest of suffering. Therefore, we believe that it is mandatory to provide sedation to awake patients before ventilation is withdrawn. Any use of sedative or narcotic analgesic medication to relieve the unwanted sensations would also reduce respiratory drive; the two are inseparable. It is a physiologic reality, then, that sedating the patient probably accelerates death by some small measure of time. However, it had been determined through multiple previous attempts to wean this patient from the ventilator that death would occur anyway, so sedating the patient would not in itself cause the death.

In Mr. Larson's case, we did not advise on the types or doses of sedatives, but we did encourage adequate sedation. We suggested that the attending physician consult with an experienced pulmonologist-intensivist on the details of ventilator withdrawal, including dosing of sedation. We acknowledge that titrating sedation is difficult when the goal is relief of suffering without deliberately inducing a respiratory arrest. Marked variability in both individual needs and drug tolerance further complicates these estimates. Ideally, the patient will be heavily sedated but will continue to maintain his or her respiratory efforts.

### Our Planning

We submitted our ethics consultation report to the team and were informed by the intern that the disconnection was to be done three days later, on 25 February 1991 at 10:00 A.M. We suggest selecting a particular time for several reasons: it allows further time to assure durability of the patient's request, and it allows the patient and family to say final goodbyes, decide who will be present, arrange last rites, and so forth; in addition, selecting a time early in the day ensures that the physician and primary nurses are available in case the patient does not die right away and needs further comfort and support. A disadvantage of setting a specific time is that any delay will be a further stress for the patient and family.

Final details were planned with the patient and the health care team. The patient requested that several members of his family be present (they wanted to be there), while others would wait in an adjoining room. The primary care team discussed who would do the disconnection and decided that the pulmonary consultant and attending staff physician would administer sedatives and disconnect the ventilator. We saw our role as ethics consultants finished.

### The Disconnection

Loving family had been present throughout Mr. Larson's stay, and their numbers increased as the time of disconnection approached. By 9 A.M., 25 February, 13 family members and close friends were at the patient's bedside awaiting the disconnection. All anticipated that this would lead to the patient's death. We were not in attendance. At 9:30 A.M., we received a call from a distraught intern telling us that the family was there and all were ready. However, both the pulmonologist and the attending physician would not be available until 5 hours later, at 3 P.M. The intern felt that she alone would have to disconnect the ventilator, something she was not technically or emotionally prepared to do and had never done before. The primary care team had not verified the pulmonary consultant's availability when the disconnection was planned. The attending physician had been called away unexpectedly and had delegated this job to the intern. We believed very strongly that this would not be an appropriate procedure for the anxious intern to do alone. Although we were both technically qualified as pulmonologist-intensivist and internist to perform the disconnection, we felt that being involved this way was beyond our role as ethics consultants. (We believe that an experienced pulmonologist-intensivist should always be involved.) Nevertheless, the patient had already waited a week while we had undertaken the seven actions outlined earlier, and we felt it would be cruel for him and his family to wait any longer. So with much trepidation, we decided that we would provide sedation and disconnect the ventilator ourselves. After this experience, we conclude that the attending physician *should* be the main player, with a pulmonologist-intensivist in attendance to provide necessary technical expertise. This is not a job for interns or inexperienced physicians.

We talked with the patient again to see if he still wanted this to be done and informed him that we would be performing the disconnection. He said yes emphatically. The family and other members of the health care team agreed. We told the patient we could not know exactly what dose of medication would be ideal and that we might err in either direction. We explained that if we judged low in our estimate, he would suffer from dyspnea. We asked his permission to reconnect the ventilator briefly if that happened, so that we could calmly administer additional medication. We would then disconnect again. He hesitated, but agreed. We again reminded him and the family that he might not die immediately. We told them that although we did not expect it, there was a slight chance he might continue to breathe for 24 hours or more. Our tests indicated he would not be able to breathe on his own, but occasionally patients live longer than we expect. If such was the case, we planned to start an intravenous drip of morphine to ensure his comfort.

A venous line was placed. We looked into the face of an alert man who we knew would soon die. Our more rational intellects told us that his disease, not us, would be the cause of his death. Deep feelings, on the other hand, were accusing us of causing death. From deep within us, feelings were speaking to us, making accusations, "You are really killing him, practicing active euthanasia, deceptively rationalizing with your intellects that there is a difference." These were not new feelings, but they were now greatly intensified as we stood there next to the patient, preparing to use syringes containing midazolam and morphine. Both are known respiratory depressants, which at high doses would be effective in active euthanasia and even at therapeutic doses would at least cause some respiratory depression and perhaps an earlier death. Nevertheless, midazolam and morphine were medically indicated to provide comfort to withdraw the ventilator in compliance with his request. We respected his right to refuse further life dependent on the ventilator. A heavy feeling of intense emotion consumed both of us as we slowly injected midazolam and morphine, watching the patient closely so we could produce the desired level of drowsiness. He reached what we thought was the correct end point, and one of us disconnected the tube to the ventilator while the other was poised at the catheter in case more medication was necessary. We stood frozen as Mr. Larson continued to take shallow but regular breaths. We felt some relief; at least we had not sedated the patient so heavily that this alone would cause his immediate death.

Within a minute or so, the patient turned slightly cyanotic and began to struggle. With trembling hands, we pushed more midazolam and morphine, reaching final total doses of 15 mg midazolam and 30 mg morphine sulfate. (These doses apply directly to this patient and are not recommended for anybody else; people differ greatly in their tolerances.) Mr. Larson seemed comfortable, breathing shallowly at a rate of 28/minute. He exchanged smiles with his daughter, who stood holding his hand across the bed. He appeared reasonably comfortable and relaxed. We both felt a great heaviness and deep sense of anxiety. To facilitate communication among the 13 friends and family, we requested further support by the patient advocate (who had also been involved throughout the earlier discussions). Several family members provided regular updates to family members in the adjoining room. His daughter, the primary nurse, the intern, and the two of us remained at his bedside. Mr. Larson did not struggle further. About 30 minutes passed, although it seemed like hours. The patient then gradually slipped into a coma. Forty-five minutes after the disconnection, his breathing became irregular and stopped. He was not attached to any monitors, which probably reduced the strain on the family during the final minutes. His heart continued to beat for several minutes, first regularly, then with pauses. We took turns listening and waited until we were certain that he had died. Fifty-three minutes after he was disconnected from the ventilator, we pronounced him dead.

Although we received grateful hugs from the family and thanks from the health care team, we were struck by the gravity of what we had done. Doubts kept creeping into our minds. We each experienced a wave of disquieting emotion, feelings that we had killed this patient who would have otherwise continued to live connected to the ventilator. We knew intellectually that he had the legal and ethical right to refuse this medical treatment, but the gravity of his decision and our participation haunted us. We returned to our immediate commitments of caring for other patients, one of us responding next to the need of a patient who wanted medical help for a pulmonary problem to prolong his life. Both of us remained preoccupied throughout the afternoon thinking about Mr. Larson and what we had done. Our respective medical careers have generally been devoted to responding to patient wishes to postpone death and to prolong life. We've seen our patients die of their various diseases, but now our acquiescence in allowing his death caused us much anguish. This anguish continued in both of us for several days. One of us sought counsel from a psychiatrist who reinforced our belief that we did the right thing, counteracting those deep feelings that somehow we had killed this patient. Gradually we came to terms with what had happened. We had been in a complicated situation in which technology was sustaining life artificially, and we had acted on this patient's choice to refuse that treatment. Our consciences were clear, but we were left feeling very impressed with how difficult it had been to honor this man's request.

It is beyond the usual role of ethics consultants to take over patient care responsibilities and actually perform ventilator withdrawal. We do not intend to make it our practice to do this because it is really the appropriate role of the care providers, who should enlist the help of a pulmonary-intensivist. We appreciate what we have learned from this unusual experience. After a period of reflection, we are no longer anxious about this decision, and we believe that we did the right thing in respecting Mr. Larson's request. Having witnessed from the bedside the suffering and the determination of this patient and his family, we feel better equipped to counsel other physicians whose patient care responsibilities will require them to grapple with similar end-of-life dilemmas.

## Note

The name of our patient was changed to protect patient confidentiality, and the family granted permission to share his story. The authors thank Bernard Lo, MD, Michael Garland, DScRel, Virginia Tilden, DNSc., and Sandy Poole for their thoughtful reviews of the original manuscript.

## The Promise
Sharon Olds

With the second drink, at the restaurant,
holding hands on the bare table,
we are at it again, renewing our promise
to kill each other. You are drinking gin,
night-blue juniper berry
dissolving in your body, I am drinking Fumé,
chewing its fragrant dirt and smoke, we are
taking on earth, we are part soil already,
and wherever we are, we are also in our
bed, fitted, naked, closely
along each other, half passed out,
after love, drifting back
and forth across the border of consciousness,
our bodies buoyant, clasped. Your hand
tightens on the table. You're a little afraid
I'll chicken out. What you do not want
is to lie in a hospital bed for a year
after a stroke, without being able
to think or die, you do not want
to be tied to a chair like your prim grandmother,
cursing. The room is dim around us,

Sharon Olds, "The Promise," *Blood, Tin, Straw.* © 1999 by Sharon Olds. Reprinted by permission of Alfred A. Knopf, Inc.

ivory globes, pink curtains
bound at the waist—and outside,
a weightless, luminous, lifted-up
summer twilight. I tell you you do not
know me if you think I will not
kill you. Think how we have floated together
eye to eye, nipple to nipple,
sex to sex, the halves of a creature
drifting up to the lip of matter
and over it—you know me from the bright, blood-
flecked delivery room, if a lion
had you in its jaws I would attack it, if the ropes
binding your soul are your own wrists, I will cut them.

## Death and Dignity: A Case of Individualized Decision Making
Timothy E. Quill

Diane was feeling tired and had a rash. A common scenario, though there was something subliminally worrisome that prompted me to check her blood count. Her hematocrit was 22, and the white-cell count was 4.3 with some metamyelocytes and unusual white cells. I wanted it to be viral, trying to deny what was staring me in the face. Perhaps in a repeated count it would disappear. I called Diane and told her it might be more serious than I had initially thought—that the test needed to be repeated and that if she felt worse, we might have to move quickly. When she pressed for the possibilities, I reluctantly opened the door to leukemia. Hearing the word seemed to make it exist. "Oh, shit!" she said. "Don't tell me that." Oh, shit! I thought, I wish I didn't have to.

Diane was no ordinary person (although no one I have ever come to know has been really ordinary). She was raised in an alcoholic family and had felt alone for much of her life. She had vaginal cancer as a young woman. Through much of her adult life, she had struggled with depression and her own alcoholism. I had come to know, respect, and admire her over the previous eight years as she confronted these problems and gradually overcame them. She was an incredibly clear, at times brutally honest, thinker and communicator. As she took control of her life, she developed a strong sense of independence and confidence. In the previous 3½ years, her hard work had paid off. She was completely abstinent from alcohol, she had established much deeper connections with her husband, college-age son, and several friends, and her business and her artistic work were blossoming. She felt she was really living fully for the first time.

Not surprisingly, the repeated blood count was abnormal, and detailed examination of the peripheral-blood smear showed myelocytes. I advised her to come into the hospital, explaining that we needed to do a bone marrow biopsy and make some decisions relatively rapidly. She came to the hospital knowing what we would find. She was terrified, angry, and sad. Although we knew the odds, we both clung to the thread of possibility that it might be something else.

The bone marrow confirmed the worst: acute myelomonocytic leukemia. In the face of this tragedy, we looked for signs of hope. This is an area of medicine in which technological intervention has been successful, with cures 25 percent of the time—long-term cures. As I probed the costs of these cures, I heard about induction chemotherapy (three weeks in the hospital, prolonged neutropenia, probable infectious complications, and hair loss; 75 percent of patients respond, 25 percent do not). For the survivors, this is followed by consolidation chemotherapy (with similar side effects; another 25 percent die, for a net survival of 50 percent). Those still alive, to have a reasonable chance of long-term survival, then need bone marrow transplantation (hospitalization for two months and whole-body irradiation, with complete killing of the bone marrow, infectious complications, and the possibility for graft-versus-host disease—with a survival of approximately 50 percent, or 25 percent of the original group). Though hematologists may argue over the exact percentages, they don't argue about the outcome of no treatment—certain death in days, weeks, or at most a few months.

Believing that delay was dangerous, our oncologist broke the news to Diane and began making plans to insert a Hickman catheter and begin induction chemotherapy that afternoon. When I saw her shortly thereafter, she was enraged at his presumption that she would want treatment, and devastated by the finality of the diagnosis. All she wanted to do was go home and be with her family. She had no further questions about treatment and in fact had decided that she wanted none. Together we lamented her tragedy and the unfairness of life. Before she left, I felt the need to be sure that she and her husband understood that there was some risk in delay, that the problem was not going to go away, and that we needed to keep considering the options over the next several days. We agreed to meet in two days.

She returned in two days with her husband and son. They had talked extensively about the problem and the options. She remained very clear about her wish not to undergo chemotherapy and to live whatever time she had left outside the hospital. As we explored her thinking further, it became clear that she was convinced she would die during the period of treatment and would suffer unspeakably in the process (from hospitalization, from lack of control over her body, from the side effects of chemotherapy, and from pain and anguish). Although I could offer support and my best effort to minimize her suffering if she chose treatment, there was no way I could say any of this would not occur. In fact, the last four patients with acute leukemia at our hospital had died very painful deaths in the hospital during various stages of treatment (a fact I did not share with her). Her family wished she would choose treatment but sadly accepted her decision. She articulated very clearly that it was she who would be experiencing all the side effects of treatment and that odds of 25 percent were not good enough for her to undergo so toxic a course of therapy, given her expectations of chemotherapy and hospitalization and the absence of a closely matched bone marrow donor. I had her repeat her understanding of the treatment, the odds, and what to expect if there were no treatment. I clarified a few misunderstandings, but she had a remarkable grasp of the options and implications.

I have been a longtime advocate of active, informed patient choice of treatment or nontreatment, and of a patient's right to die with as much control and dignity as possible. Yet there was something about her giving up a 25 percent chance of long-term survival in favor of almost certain death that disturbed me. I had seen Diane fight and use her considerable inner resources to overcome alcoholism and depression, and I half expected her to change her mind over the next week. Since the window of time in which effective treatment can be initiated is rather narrow, we met several times that week. We obtained a second hematology consultation and talked at length about the meaning and implications of treatment and nontreatment. She talked to a psychologist she had seen in the past. I gradually understood the decision from her perspective and became convinced that it was the right decision for her. We arranged for home hospice care (although at that time Diane felt reasonably well, was active, and looked healthy), left the door open for her to change her mind, and tried to anticipate how to keep her comfortable in the time she had left.

Just as I was adjusting to her decision, she opened up another area that would stretch me profoundly. It was extraordinarily important to Diane to maintain control of herself and her own dignity during the time remaining to her. When this was no longer possible, she clearly wanted to die. As a former director of a hospice program, I know how to use pain medicines to keep patients comfortable and lessen suffering. I explained the philosophy of comfort care, which I strongly believe in. Although Diane understood and appreciated this, she had known of people lingering in what was called relative comfort, and she wanted no part of it. When the time came, she wanted to take her life in the least painful way possible. Knowing of her desire for independence and her decision to stay in control, I thought this request made perfect sense. I acknowledged and explored this wish but also thought that it was out of the realm of currently accepted medical practice and that it was more than I could offer or promise. In our discussion, it became clear that preoccupation with her fear of a lingering death would interfere with Diane's getting the most out of the time she had left until she found a safe way to ensure her death. I feared the effects of a violent death on her family, the consequences of an ineffective suicide that would leave her lingering in precisely the state she dreaded so much, and the possibility that a family member would be forced to assist her, with all the legal and personal repercussions that would follow. She discussed this at length with her family. They believed that they should respect her choice. With this in mind, I told Diane that information was available from the Hemlock Society that might be helpful to her.

A week later she phoned me with a request for barbiturates for sleep. Since I knew that this was an essential ingredient in a Hemlock Society suicide, I asked her to come to the office to talk things over. She was more than willing to protect me by participating in a superficial conversation about her insomnia, but it was important to me to know how she planned to use the drugs and to be sure that she was not in despair or overwhelmed in a way that might color her judgment. In our discussion, it was apparent that she was having trouble sleeping, but it was also evident that the security of having enough barbiturates available to commit suicide when and if the time came would leave her secure enough to live fully and concentrate on the present. It was clear that she was not despondent and that in fact she was making deep, personal connections with her family and close friends. I made sure that she knew how to use the barbiturates for sleep, and also that she knew the amount needed to commit suicide. We agreed to meet regularly, and she promised to meet with me before taking her life, to ensure that all other avenues had been exhausted. I wrote the prescription with an uneasy feeling about the boundaries I was exploring—spiritual, legal, professional, and personal. Yet I also felt strongly that I was setting her free to get the most out of the time she had left, and to maintain dignity and control on her own terms until her death.

The next several months were very intense and important for Diane. Her son stayed home from college, and they were able to be with one another and say much that had not been said earlier. Her husband did his work at home so that he and Diane could spend more time together. She spent time with her closest friends. I had her come into the hospital for a conference with our residents, at which she illustrated in a most profound and personal way the importance of informed decision making, the right to refuse treatment, and the extraordinarily personal effects of illness and interaction with the medical system. There were emotional and physical hardships as well. She had periods of intense sadness and anger. Several times she became very weak, but she received transfusions as an outpatient and responded with marked improvement of symptoms. She had two serious infections that responded surprisingly well to empirical courses of oral antibiotics. After three tumultuous months, there were two weeks of relative calm and well-being, and fantasies of a miracle began to surface.

Unfortunately, we had no miracle. Bone pain, weakness, fatigue, and fevers began to dominate her life. Although the hospice workers, family members, and I tried our best to minimize the suffering and promote comfort, it was clear that the end was approaching. Diane's immediate future held what she feared the most—increasing discomfort, dependence, and hard choices between pain and sedation. She called up her closest friends and asked them to come over to say goodbye, telling them that she would be leaving soon. As we had agreed, she let me know as well. When we met, it was clear that she knew what she was doing, that she was sad and frightened to be leaving, but that she would be even more terrified to stay and suffer. In our tearful goodbye, she promised a reunion in the future at her favorite spot on the edge of Lake Geneva, with dragons swimming in the sunset.

Two days later her husband called to say that Diane had died. She had said her final goodbyes to her husband and son that morning, and asked them to leave her alone for an hour. After an hour, which must have seemed an eternity, they found her on the couch, lying very still and covered by her favorite shawl. There was no sign of struggle. She seemed to be at peace. They called me for advice about how to proceed. When I arrived at their house, Diane indeed seemed peaceful. Her husband and son were quiet. We talked about what a remarkable person she had been. They seemed to have no doubts about the course she had chosen or about their cooperation, although the unfairness of her illness and the finality of her death were overwhelming to us all.

I called the medical examiner to inform him that a hospice patient had died. When asked about the cause of death, I said, "Acute leukemia." He said that was fine and that we should call a funeral director. Although acute leukemia was the truth, it was not the whole story. Yet any mention of suicide would have given rise to a police investigation and probably brought the arrival of an ambulance crew for resuscitation. Diane would have become a "coroner's case," and the decision to perform an autopsy would have been made at the discretion of the medical examiner. The family or I could have been subject to criminal prosecution, and I to professional review, for our roles in support of Diane's choices. Although I truly believe that the family and I gave her the best care possible, allowing her to define her limits and directions as much as possible, I am not sure the law, society, or the medical profession would agree. So I said "acute leukemia" to protect all of us, to protect Diane from an invasion into her past and her body, and to continue to shield society from the knowledge of the degree of suffering that people often undergo in the process of dying. Suffering can be lessened to some extent, but in no way eliminated or made benign, by the careful intervention of a competent, caring physician, given current social constraints.

Diane taught me about the range of help I can provide if I know people well and if I allow them to say what they really want. She taught me about life, death, and honesty and about taking charge and facing tragedy squarely when it strikes. She taught me that I can take small risks for people that I really know and care about. Although I did not assist in her suicide directly, I helped indirectly to make it possible, successful, and relatively painless. Although I know we have measures to help control pain and lessen suffering, to think that people do not suffer in the process of dying is an illusion. Prolonged dying can occasionally be peaceful, but more often the role of the physician and family is limited to lessening but not eliminating severe suffering.

I wonder how many families and physicians secretly help patients over the edge into death in the face of such severe suffering. I wonder how many severely ill or dying patients secretly take their lives, dying alone in despair. I wonder whether the image of Diane's final aloneness will persist in the minds of her family, or if they will remember more the intense, meaningful months they had together before she died. I wonder whether Diane struggled in that last hour, and whether the Hemlock Society's way of death by suicide is the most benign. I wonder why Diane, who gave so much to so many of us, had to be alone for the last hour of her life. I wonder whether I will see Diane again, on the shore of Lake Geneva at sunset, with dragons swimming on the horizon.

## Correspondence
## Death and Dignity: The Case of Diane

*To the Editor*: I am a retired general surgeon essentially quadriplegic and dependent on a respirator because of advanced amyotrophic lateral sclerosis.

Timothy Quill's Sounding Board article (March 7 issue)[1] was beautifully written and quite obviously reflects the thinking of a sensitive, caring health professional. I fully agree with the decision made, the rationale for that decision, and the action taken.

Who better than the individual patient can decide when the burdens that illness imposes on oneself, one's family, and society can no longer be justified by any possible contribution to the well-being of anyone? Transient extremes of depression are correctly resisted by all; nonetheless, to the patient, there has to be an acceptable reason for carrying on.

Of course I agree that the decision to seek death must be challenged by the medical profession and the family, but if no valid rationale can be offered for sustained existence, what then? Can the profession justify simply walking away from the problem? I think not.

Why should a spouse or child or a dedicated health professional be subjected to the threat of a legal proceeding for easing the suffering of a desperately ill person who consciously and rationally asks that the anguish be ended?

When my continued survival is no longer meaningful (to me), I hope that a caring physician will make the transition as easy as possible. I realize that some health professionals will find it impossible to do this, but I hope that they and society will understand the true compassion for their patients'

Correspondence: Response to "Death and Dignity: The Case of Diane," from *New England Journal of Medicine*, vol. 325, 201–203. © 1991 by the Massachusetts Medical Society. Reprinted by permission of the publisher.

suffering that motivates the physicians who do help those in need. And I would hope that this understanding will lead to the elimination of unwarranted legal constraints when patient, family, and physician all concur.

Stewart A. King, M.D.

27 Harbor Road, Darien, CT 06820

*To the Editor:* . . . Dr. Quill provided his patient with exactly what was lacking in the more notorious cases involving Dr. Jack Kevorkian and the anonymous author of "It's Over, Debbie":[2] comprehensive medical care, with deep concern for the patient's well-being and respect for her choices. The debate concerning euthanasia and assisted suicide will continue, but we now have one additional reference point: a conscientious physician providing excellent medical care.

Jack P. Freer, M.D.

Millard Fillmore Hospital, Buffalo, NY 14209

*To the Editor:* Dr. Quill's suggestion that physicians may frequently engage in assisting suicides is incorrect. In most states, as in his own, assisting suicide is illegal. It is never the role of a physician to help a patient perform such an act. In fact, it is the role of a physician to prevent suicide attempts whenever there is a possibility that they may occur. In this situation, as in other situations in which physicians are faced with the threatened death of their patients due to illness, it is the role of the physician to apply his or her knowledge, skill, and caring to save lives. . . .

Lisa J. Cardo, M.D.

Albert Einstein College of Medicine, Bronx, NY 10467

*To the Editor:* . . . It should be made clear that assisted suicide is not a part of hospice care. The standards of the National Hospice Organization specifically state that hospices affirm life and neither hasten nor postpone death.[3] Moreover, at its 1990 annual meeting, the organization adopted a resolution that rejected the practice of voluntary euthanasia and assisted suicide in the care of the terminally ill. . . .

Michael H. Levy, M.D., Ph.D.

National Hospice Organization, Arlington, VA 22209

*To the Editor:* As I reflect on my mother's decision to choose palliative care in the presence of an acute and rapidly progressing malignant melanoma, and on her physician's insistence on chemotherapy and lack of concern for her wish to spend her last days in control of her life without pain, I am saddened that her health care providers lacked the courage that Dr. Quill displayed in the treatment of his patient Diane. . . .

Joshua A. Bloomstone

Albert Einstein College of Medicine, Bronx, NY 10467

*To the Editor*: . . . A one-in-four chance of living is a fighting chance for a relatively young woman with as full a life as Dr. Quill describes. Any physician should be reluctant to let a patient like this forgo such an opportunity for life, without applying all his or her powers of persuasion and personally invoking the love of family and friends and the expertise and support of a psychiatrist, the patient's nurses, a clergyperson or patient advocate, a social worker, and maybe a patient or two who risked the uncertainty of treatment in similar circumstances. An intense demonstration of caring, listening, and communication might well have helped this woman face her crisis differently or at least with greater solace. . . .

Michael T. Ross, M.D.

3997 Raintree Drive, Troy, MI 48083

*To the Editor*: The fact that Diane elected to die alone to protect her family from possible criminal charges represents a gross failure on the part of society in general and a failure on the part of us as physicians. How poignant it is that Diane could not have spent her final moments in the presence of a loved one.

Here in Washington State, 223,000 voters have signed Initiative 119—the "death with dignity" initiative. If passed by the general electorate in November, it will expand our existing Natural Death Act, allowing the withdrawal of certain measures—i.e., the administration of fluids and nutrition—in specific cases. It also broadens the definition of "terminal" illness to include irreversible coma and a persistent vegetative state.

More controversially, Initiative 119 would allow a terminally ill patient to request help in dying from a physician who is willing to provide it. Safeguards would include the requirements that the patient be terminally ill and expected to die within six months, as deemed by two physicians; that the patient be a mentally competent adult; and that the request must be made in writing and witnessed by two persons. The provision for help

in dying is voluntary in every respect: no one would be required to participate on any level, as patient or as provider.

Linda Gromko, M.D.

Neil F. Thorlakson, M.D.

Physicians for Yes on Initiative 119, Bellevue, WA 98004

*To the Editor*: Dr. Quill was right to question "whether the Hemlock Society's way of death by suicide is the most benign." Diane's self-deliverance
was a second-best option because the law does not yet permit the best
way.

Diane should have been able to die in the presence of loved ones, and
Dr. Quill ought to have been allowed to administer the drug and monitor
its effect....

Derek Humphry

National Hemlock Society, Eugene, OR 97440

*To the Editor*: That a physician would assist a patient in ending her life in
the face of unremitting disability and a terminal disease is not unusual.[4]
In discussing bioethics with groups of physicians, I have rarely found a
primary care clinician who has not helped a patient to die who was de-
sirous of ending intolerable pain or disability in the midst of a terminal
disease. Most of these clinicians, however, take a more circumspect approach than Dr. Quill, prescribing narcotics or barbiturates with the explicit caveat, "Don't take this many, or it will kill you."...

Kenneth V. Iserson, M.D.

University of Chicago, Chicago, IL 60637

*To the Editor*: ... Dr. Quill's eight-year acquaintance with his patient is
only partly reassuring. The most disturbing cases of assisted suicide are
those in which a physician with little familiarity with a patient serves
only to provide an instrument of peaceful death. It is hard to doubt Dr.
Quill's fondness for his patient. What is disturbing is that this association may have become a personal friendship that threatened even the
limited impartiality that would be present in a more detached professional relationship.

Physicians themselves, who feel powerless in the face of terminal illnesses in their patients, behave in various ways. Some project their own
hopelessness onto the patient, thus sanctioning or even unwittingly encouraging an assisted suicide. Others, sharing helplessness about the

prognosis, collude with the patient to wrest control of death from the fatal disease. Quill's account states that his patient had a history of depression and alcoholism. He provides only minimal assurance that he tried to determine that she was not overwhelmed or in despair. Did he obtain the consultation of a more detached colleague or psychiatrist to determine whether the patient was clinically depressed? Likewise, it is important to know that Quill himself was not despairing. Did he speak with other trusted colleagues or friends about his plans, or did he arrive at his decision to assist a suicide in his own mind—alone, helpless, frightened of either choice he would make, as he watched a friend succumb to an illness he could not control? . . .

Peter M. Marzuk, M.D.

Cornell University Medical College, New York, NY 10021

*To the Editor*: The case of Diane is a "hard case" for those who would continue the current policy forbidding physicians to assist patients in committing suicide, because the patient had the best of care and the best of family support; decided on her own that the continued suffering from pain and disability and the tragedy of fatal illness were more than she cared to endure; and presumably, determined for herself the time and manner of dying. The physician's role was, at most, one of making this course possible while trying to offer and improve on other alternatives. Lawyers often note that "hard cases make bad law."

Few patients die in such supportive surroundings. Few have a physician who is so thoughtful and skilled or a family that has comparable emotional and financial resources. Instead, pain control and emotional support are given low priority in health care. Under the current health care "system," most of us will die in old age, with family scattered and resources used up, in the care of anonymous providers with limited skills and commitment. The pressures to allow active euthanasia arise largely from the wholesale inadequacy of the health care and legal systems to care for chronically ill and disabled persons who are slowly dying. These pressures do not arise from the few, like Diane, who have available all that can be done and find it still so inadequate that they prefer an earlier, self-administered death.

If we had a system of care that ensured housing and food, compassion, symptomatic relief, family support, and self-determination by the patient (short of assisted suicide), then the question of allowing help so that suicide would be easy and reliable would be important and interesting. Now, in a system that routinely fails in each of the above functions, the risks of adopting a public policy allowing physicians to assist in suicide (or any form of active euthanasia) are simply too great. This society is too likely to accept the death of sufferers rather than the development of effective systems of care and support.

Joanne Lynn, M.D.
Joan Teno, M.D.
George Washington University, Washington, DC 20037

To the Editor: . . . The prohibition against assisted suicide may serve the salutary purpose of ensuring that an act that ought to require courage and compassion does not become routine. Eliminating that prohibition would eliminate the need for courage and would not instill the need for compassion. On the contrary, it makes the proliferation of suicide machines and the scenario symbolized by Debbie's fate[5] more likely than the one involving Dr. Quill and Diane.

As we wonder with Dr. Quill about what Diane's death means and ought to mean to the rest of us, we should wonder whether all change is progress and whether legalizing assisted suicide, though it may seem the next step in advancing self-determination for patients, would actually be a grave misstep. And as we wonder about whether we might make death easier for people like Diane, we ought to ask what it says about us that we spend so much time improving the fate of those who have access to a caring physician and so little addressing the gruesome fate that awaits those who have no doctor and little say in how they live or die.

Giles R. Scofield, J.D.
Cleveland Clinic Foundation, Cleveland, OH 44195

To the Editor: . . . Most cultures in history have outlawed euthanasia because they found, presumably through experience, that it was terribly destructive of the community and of positive human values. But we modern physicians are facing a time when our leading ethicists are questioning both the Hippocratic ethic and the basic ethical traditions of the West.[6] We see a "quite extraordinary confusion over elementary questions of morality—as if an instinct in such matters were truly the last thing to be taken for granted in our time."[7]

Right now, we are being encouraged to legalize "physician-assisted suicide." But once we view death as a "therapeutic treatment," the slide down the slippery slope is inevitable.[8] What comes next (if the Dutch euthanasia program is an example)[9] is euthanasia for the chronically ill patient without a terminal illness. And since some modern bioethicists have decided that the profoundly retarded and the severely brain-damaged should not be considered persons[10] (that is, as having civil rights), I am sure that we will soon be reading that it is ethical and compassionate to allow these "empty shells of human beings" the "right to die."

It is often argued that we physicians are too humane to abuse the "privilege" of euthanasia. But the lesson of the Holocaust is the banality of evil:[11] in a time of moral confusion, good people can be corrupted so that they do not recognize what is evil; others know certain deeds are wrong but do them anyway, since society has told them these deeds are correct and legal; and the majority keep silence.

N. K. O'Connor, M.D.
884 First St., Nanty Glo, PA 15943

*To the Editor*: Quill describes how he provided barbiturates to a suicidal terminally ill patient and then concealed the probable cause of death from the local medical examiner. Although assisting a suicide treads the boundaries of medical ethics, we are more concerned about the deliberate misrepresentation of the cause of death. Dr. Quill believes that recording acute leukemia as the cause of death involved a partial "truth." Although it would require an autopsy and toxicologic confirmation, forensic pathologists and the law would classify the cause of death as barbiturate poisoning and the manner of death as suicide.

Kurt B. Nolte, M.D.
Ross E. Zumwalt, M.D.
Office of the Medical Investigator, Albuquerque, NM 87131

*To the Editor*: I salute Dr. Quill on several counts. First, he stayed with Diane. Too many in our profession seem to have forgotten how important it is to stand with our patients when the outcome is in doubt, when the right course is ambiguous, when we cannot display our diagnostic brilliance and our therapeutic power. That choice alone takes courage. Second, he wrestled with Diane's particular needs, even though that effort took him far into uncharted waters as he probed for an ethical response to her dilemma. He affirmed her unique identity and proved himself to be *her* doctor. Third, he found the incredible mettle to write about it and to sign his essay, exposing himself to endless second-guessing and, perhaps, recriminations. I admire him for all these reasons, quite apart from whether I agree with the course he took. (For the record, I do.)

Robert D. Mauro, M.D.
University of Colorado School of Medicine, Denver, CO 80262

*To the Editor*: At a time when ethical and practice decisions concerning dialysis, artificial feeding, intubation, and cardiopulmonary resuscitation are made by a group or bureaucratic process, it is refreshing to know that one patient and one physician can still decide the process and outcome of medical care.

David R. Perera, M.D., M.P.H.
Group Health Medical Center, Seattle, WA 98112

*The above letters were referred to Dr. Quill, who offers the following reply*:

*To the Editor*: Dr. King eloquently articulates the aspirations of a severely ill, courageous person who still finds meaning in his struggle but hopes for an easy transition to death when his fight for life loses meaning. Struggling with such persons to continue to find meaning in life and dignity in death is one of our highest callings as physicians.

Dr. Cardo suggests that the physician's role is only to save life. In dying persons, relieving symptoms, enhancing control, and preserving dignity clearly take precedence over saving life. These values underlie the hospice philosophy. Although intensive comfort care can adequately lessen the suffering of most dying persons, some continue to suffer intolerably in spite of our best efforts, and request aid in dying. Though the National Hospice Organization opposes such aid, it is not clear what approach it advocates in these troubling circumstances.

I agree with Dr. Ross that a one-in-four chance of life is worth fighting for and that the choice of forgoing treatment should not be accepted passively by the physician. Yet, the three of every four patients who experience difficult deaths during some phase of leukemia treatment should not be dismissed in the discussion. Patients need to be fully informed rather than powerfully persuaded by their health care providers.

Drs. Gromko and Thorlakson and Mr. Humphry capture the greatest tragedy in Diane's story—that she had to die alone to protect her family and physician from legal prosecution. Initiative 119 in Washington State is a public referendum to decide whether terminally ill persons should have the right to request help in dying openly from their physicians. By requiring a direct, honest exchange between physician and patient, verified by others, such a law would prevent the indirect, ambiguous guidance by physicians that is described by Dr. Iserson, and the isolation and despair feared by Dr. Marzuk. Diane's family, my trusted colleagues, and her former psychologist were all quietly consulted, and agreed that her choices were not distorted. Under Initiative 119, Diane would not have had to be secretive about her intentions or alone at the end.

I agree with Drs. Lynn and Teno and with Mr. Scofield that the health care system is woefully inadequate in meeting the basic needs of housing, food, and access to medical care, but to deny self-determination to hopelessly ill persons until these systematic inadequacies can be solved only compounds the injustice. The fears of Dr. O'Connor about the "slippery slope"—that society will abuse assisted suicide or euthanasia to solve the social problems of the weak and powerless—can be allayed by restricting aid in dying to competent, terminally ill persons who clearly request it. Our current slippery slope denies many persons a dignified death and compels them to suffer without personal meaning or hope of recovery.

Drs. Nolte and Zumwalt are concerned about the accuracy and completeness of the death certificate. Reporting the possibility of a barbiturate overdose to the medical examiner would have led to the arrival of an ambulance crew for potential cardiopulmonary resuscitation, extensive interrogation of the family, and an unwanted and meaningless autopsy. Allowing the privacy of Diane's family to be invaded after struggling to find meaning to her illness and death seemed morally wrong.

Timothy E. Quill, M.D.

Genesee Hospital, Rochester, NY 14607

### Notes

1   Quill TE. Death and dignity—a case of individualized decision making. *N Engl J Med* 1991; 324:691–4.

2   It's over, Debbie. *JAMA* 1988; 259:272.

3   *Standards of a hospice program of care.* Arlington, Va.: National Hospice Organization, 1987.

4   Wanzer SH, Federman DD, Adelstein SJ, et al. The physician's responsibility toward hopelessly ill patients: a second look. *N Engl J Med* 1989; 320:844–9.

5 It's over, Debbie. *JAMA* 1988; 259:272.

6 Pellegrino ED. Medical ethics: entering the post-Hippocratic era. *J Am Board Fam Pract* 1988; 1:230–7.

7 Arendt H. *Eichmann in Jerusalem: a report on the banality of evil.* Rev. ed. New York: Penguin Books, 1977:295.

8 Lifton RJ. *The Nazi doctors: medical killing and the psychology of genocide.* New York: Basic Books, 1986:14, 45–79.

9 Dutch in agonizing debate over voluntary euthanasia. *Pittsburgh Press.* July 31, 1989:1.

10 Fletcher J. Indicators of humanhood: a tentative profile of man. Hastings Cent Rep 1972; 2(5):1–4.

11 Arendt H. *Eichmann in Jerusalem: a report on the banality of evil.*

## Doctor, I Want to Die. Will You Help Me?
Timothy E. Quill

It had been 18 months since a 67-year-old retired man whose main joy in life was his two grandchildren was diagnosed with inoperable lung cancer. An arduous course of chemotherapy helped him experience a relatively good year where he was able to remain independent, babysitting regularly for his grandchildren.

Recent tests revealed multiple new bony metastases. An additional round of chemotherapy and radiation provided little relief. By summer, pain and fatigue became unrelenting. He was no longer able to tolerate, much less care for, his grandchildren. His wife of 45 years devoted herself to his care and support. Nonetheless, his days felt empty and his nights were dominated by despair about the future. Though he was treated with modern pain control methods, his severe bone pain required daily choices between pain and sedation. Death was becoming less frightening than life itself.

A particularly severe thigh pain led to the roentgenogram that showed circumferential destruction of his femur. Attempting to preserve his ability to walk, he consented to the placement of a metal plate. Unfortunately, the bone was too brittle to support the plate. He would never walk again.

One evening in the hospital after his wife had just left, his physician sat down to talk. The pain was "about the same," and the new sleep medication "helped a little." He seemed quiet and distracted. When asked what was on his mind, he looked directly at his doctor and said, "Doctor, I want to die. Will you help me?"

Timothy E. Quill, "Doctor, I Want to Die. Will You Help Me?," from *Journal of the American Medical Association*, vol. 270, 225–228. © 1993 by the American Medical Association. Reprinted by permission of the publisher.

Such requests are dreaded by physicians. There is a desperate directness that makes sidestepping the question very difficult, if not impossible. Often, we successfully avoid hearing about the inner turmoil faced by our terminally ill patients—what is happening to the person who has the disease. Yet, sometimes requests for help in dying still surface from patients with strong wills, or out of desperation when there is nowhere else to turn. Though comfort care (i.e., medical care using a hospice philosophy) provides a humane alternative to traditional medical care of the dying,[1-7] it does not always provide guidance for how to approach those rare patients who continue to suffer terribly in spite of our best efforts.

This essay explores what dying patients might be experiencing when they make such requests and offers potential physician responses. Such discussions are by no means easy for clinicians, for they may become exposed to forms and depths of suffering with which they are unfamiliar and to which they do not know how to respond. They may also fear being asked to violate their own moral standards or having to turn down someone in desperate need. Open exploration of requests for physician-assisted death can be fundamental to the humane care of a dying person, because no matter how terrifying and unresolvable their suffering appears, at least they are no longer alone with it. It also frequently opens avenues of "help" that were not anticipated and that do not involve active assistance in dying.

"Doctor, I want to die" and "Will you help me?" constitute both a statement and a query that must each be independently understood and explored. The initial response, rather than a yes or no based on assumptions about the patient's intent and meaning, might be something like: "Of course, I will try to help you, but first I need to understand your wish and your suffering, and then we can explore how I can help." Rather than shying away from the depths of suffering, follow-up questions might include, "What is the worst part?" or "What is your biggest fear?"

### The Wish to Die

Transient yearnings for death as an escape from suffering are extremely common among patients with incurable, relentlessly progressive medical illnesses.[8-10] They are not necessarily signs of a major psychiatric disorder, nor are they likely to be fully considered requests for a physician-assisted death. Let us explore some of their potential meanings through a series of case vignettes.

### Tired of Acute Medical Treatment

A 55-year-old woman with very aggressive breast cancer found her tumor to be repeatedly recurring over the previous 6 months. The latest instance signaled another failure of chemotherapy. When her doctor was proposing a new round of experimental therapy, she said, "I wish I were dead." By exploring her statement, the physician learned that the patient felt strongly she was not going to get better and that she could not fathom the prospect of more chemotherapy with its attendant side effects. She wanted to spend what time she had left at home. He also learned that she did not want to die at that moment. A discussion about changing the goals of treatment from cure to comfort ensued, and a treatment plan was developed that exchanged chemotherapy for symptom-relieving treatments. The patient was relieved by this change in focus, and she was able to spend her last month at home with her family on a hospice program.

Comfort care can guide a caring and humane approach to the last phase of life by directing its energy to relieving the patients' suffering with the same intensity and creativity that traditional medical care usually devotes to treating the underlying disease.[1-7] When comprehensively applied, in either a hospice program or any other setting, comfort care can help ensure a dignified, individualized death for most patients.

### Unrecognized or Undertreated Physical Symptoms

A stoical 85-year-old farmer with widely metastatic prostate cancer was cared for in his home with the help of a hospice program. Everyone marveled at his dry wit and engaging nature as he courageously faced death. He was taking very little medication and always said he was "fine." Everyone loved to visit with him, and his stories about life on the farm were legendary. As he became more withdrawn and caustic, people became concerned, but when he said he wished he were dead, there was a panic. All the guns on the farm were hidden and plans for a psychiatric hospitalization were entertained. When his "wish for death" was fully explored, it turned out that he was living with excruciating pain, but not telling anyone because he feared becoming "addicted" to narcotics. After a long discussion about pain-relieving principles, the patient agreed to try a regular, around-the-clock dosage of a long-acting narcotic with "as needed" doses as requested. In a short time, his pain was under better control, he again began to engage his family and visitors, and he no longer wanted to die.

For the remainder of his life, the physical symptoms that developed were addressed in a timely way, and he died a relatively peaceful death surrounded by his family.

Though not all physical symptoms can be relieved by the creative application of comfort care, most can be improved or at least made tolerable. New palliative techniques have been developed that can ameliorate most types of physical pain, provided they are applied without unnecessary restraint. One must be sure that unrelieved symptoms are not the result of ignorance about or inadequate trials of available medical treatments, or the result of exaggerated patient or physician fears about addiction or about indirectly hastening death. Experts who can provide formal or informal consultation in pain control and in palliative care are available in most major cities and extensive literature is available.[11-14]

### Emergent Psychosocial Problems

A 70-year-old retired woman with chronic leukemia that had become acute and had not responded to treatment was sent home on a home hospice program. She was prepared to die, and all of her physicians felt that she would "not last more than a few weeks." She had lived alone in the past, but her daughter took a leave of absence from work to care for her mother for her last few days or weeks. Ironically (though not necessarily surprisingly), the mother stabilized at home. Two months later, outwardly comfortable and symptom-free under the supportive watch of her daughter, she began to focus on wanting to die. When asked to elaborate, she initially discussed her fatigue and her lack of a meaningful future. She then confided that she hated being a burden on her daughter—that her daughter had children who needed her and a job that was beginning to cause serious strain. The daughter had done her best to protect her mother from these problems, but she became aware of them anyway. A family meeting where the problems were openly discussed resulted in a compromise where the mother was admitted to a nursing facility where comfort care was offered, and the daughter visited every other weekend. Though the mother ideally would have liked to stay at home, she accepted this solution and was transferred to an inpatient unit where she lived for two more months before dying with her daughter at her side.

Requests for help in dying can emanate from unrecognized or evolving psychosocial problems.[15] Sometimes these problems can be alleviated by having a family meeting, by arranging a temporary "respite" admission to a health care facility, or by consulting a social worker for some advice about finances and available services. Other psychosocial problems may be more intractable, for example, in a family that was not functioning well prior to the patient's illness or when a dominating family member tries to influence care in a direction that appears contrary to the patient's wishes or best interest. Many patients have no family and no financial resources. The current paucity of inpatient hospices and nursing facilities capable of providing comfort care and the inadequate access to health care in general in the United States often mean that dying patients who need the most help and support are forced to fend for themselves and often die by themselves. The health care reimbursement system is primarily geared toward acute medical care, but not terminal care, so the physician may be the only potential advocate and support that some dying patients have.

### Spiritual Crisis

A 42-year-old woman who was living at home with advanced acquired immunodeficiency syndrome (AIDS) began saying that she wished she were dead. She was a fundamentalist Christian who at the time of her diagnosis wondered, "Why would God do this to me?" She eventually found meaning in the possibility that God was testing her strength, and that this was her "cross to bear." Though she continued to regularly participate in church activities over the five years after her initial diagnosis, she never confided in her minister or church friends about her diagnosis. Her statements about wishing she were dead frightened her family, and they forced her to visit her doctor. When asked to elaborate on her wish, she raged against her church, her preacher, and her God, stating she found her disease humiliating and did not want to be seen in the end states of AIDS where everyone would know. She had felt more and more alone with these feelings, until they burst open. Once the feelings were acknowledged and understood, it was clear that they defied simple solution. She was clearly and legitimately angry, but not depressed. She had no real interest in taking her own life. She was eventually able to find a fundamentalist minister from a different church with an open mind about AIDS who helped her find some spiritual consolation.

The importance of the physician's role as witness and support cannot be overemphasized. Sharing feelings of spiritual betrayal and uncertainty with an empathetic listener can be the first step toward healing. At least isolation is taken out of the doubt and despair. The physician must listen and try to fully understand the problem before making any attempt to help the patient achieve spiritual resolution. Medically experienced clergy are available in many communities who can explore spiritual issues with dying patients of many faiths so that isolation can be further lessened and potential for reconnection with one's religious roots enhanced.

## Clinical Depression

A 60-year-old man with a recently diagnosed recurrence of his non-Hodgkin's lymphoma became preoccupied with wanting to die. Though he had a long remission after his first course of chemotherapy, he had recently gone through a divorce and felt he could not face more treatment. In exploring his wishes, it was evident he was preoccupied with the death of his father, who experienced an agonizing death filled with severe pain and agitation. He had a strong premonition that the same thing would happen to him, and he was not sleeping because of this preoccupation. He appeared withdrawn and was not able to fully understand and integrate his options and the odds of treatment directed at his lymphoma, the likelihood that comfort care would prevent a death like his father's, or his doctor's promise to work with him to find acceptable solutions. Though he was thinking seriously of suicide, he did not have a plan and therefore was treated intensively as an outpatient by his internist and a psychotherapist. He accepted the idea that he was depressed, but also wanted assurances that all possibilities could be explored after a legitimate trial of treatment for depression. He responded well to a combination of psychotherapy and medication. He eventually underwent acute treatment directed at his lymphoma that unfortunately did not work. He then requested hospice care and seemed comfortable and engaged in his last months. As death was imminent, his symptoms remained relatively well controlled, and he was not overtly depressed. He died alone while his family was out of the house. Since his recently filled prescription bottles were all empty, it may have been a drug overdose (presumably to avoid an end like his father's), though no note or discussion accompanied the act.

Whenever a severely ill person begins to talk about wanting to die and begins to seriously consider taking his or her own life, the question of clinical depression appropriately arises.[16] This can be a complex and delicate determination because most patients who are near death with unrelenting suffering are very sad, if not clinically depressed. The epidemiologic literature associating terminal illness and suicide assumes that all such acts arise from unrecognized and/or untreated psychiatric disorders,[17-19] yet there is a growing clinical literature suggesting that some of these suicides may be rational.[2,16,20-25]

Two fundamental questions must be answered before suicide can be considered rational in such settings: (1) Is the patient able to fully understand his or her disease, prognosis, and treatment alternatives (i.e., is the decision rational), and (2) is the patient's depression reversible, given the limitations imposed by his illness, in a way that would substantially alter the circumstances? It is vital not to overnormalize (e.g., "Anyone would be depressed under such circumstances") or to reflexively define the request as a sign of psychopathology. Each patient's dilemma must be fully explored. Consultation with an experienced psychiatrist can be helpful when there is doubt, as can a trial of grief counseling, crisis intervention, or antidepressant medications if a potentially reversible depression is present and the patient has time and strength to participate.

### Unrelenting, Intolerable Suffering

The man with widely metastatic lung cancer described in the introduction felt that his life had become a living hell with no acceptable options. His doctors agreed that all effective medical options to treat his cancer had been exhausted. Physical activity and pride in his body had always been a central part of who he was. Now, with a pathologic fracture in his femur that could not be repaired, he would not even be able to walk independently. He also had to make daily trade-offs between pain, sedation, and other side effects. At the insistence of his doctor, he had several visits with a psychiatrist who found his judgment to be fully rational. Death did not appear imminent, and his condition could only get worse. Even on a hospice program, with experts doing their best to help address his medical, social, personal, and spiritual concerns, he felt trapped, yearning for death. He saw his life savings from 45 years of work rapidly depleting. His family offered additional personal and financial resources. They wanted him to live, but having witnessed the last months of progressive disability, loss, and pain, with no relief in sight other than death, they respected his wishes and slowly began to advocate on his behalf. "We appreciate your efforts to keep him comfortable, but for him this is not comfortable and it is not living. Will you help him?"

Physicians who have made a commitment to shepherd their patients through the dying process find themselves in a predicament. They can acknowledge that comfort care is sometimes far less than ideal, but it is the best that they can offer, or they can consider making an exception to the prohibition against physician-assisted death, with its inherent personal and professional risks. Compassionate physicians differ widely on their approach to this dilemma,[20-24,26-29] though most would likely agree with an open discussion with a patient who raises the issue and an extensive search for alternatives.

Clinical criteria have been proposed to guide physicians who find assisted suicide a morally acceptable avenue of last resort:[25] (1) the patient must, of his or her own free will and at his or her own initiative, clearly and repeatedly request to die rather than continue suffering; (2) the patient's judgment must not be distorted; (3) the patient must have a condition that is incurable and associated with severe, unrelenting, intolerable suffering; (4) the physician must ensure that the patient's suffering and the request are not the result of inadequate comfort care; (5) physician-assisted suicide should only be carried out in the context of a meaningful doctor-patient relationship;[22] (6) consultation with another physician who is experienced in comfort care is required; and (7) clear documentation to support each condition above should be required (if and when such a process becomes openly sanctioned). It is not the purpose of this essay to review the policy implications of formally accepting these criteria or of maintaining current prohibitions.[20-29] Instead, it is to encourage and guide clinicians on both sides of the issue to openly explore the potential meanings of a patient's request for help in dying and to search as broadly as possible for acceptable responses that are tailored to the individual patient.

### The Request for Help in Dying

Dying patients need more than prescriptions for narcotics or referrals to hospice programs from their physicians. They need a personal guide and counselor through the dying process—someone who will unflinchingly help them face both the medical and the personal aspects of dying, whether it goes smoothly or it takes the physician into unfamiliar, untested ground. Dying patients do not have the luxury of choosing not to undertake the journey, or of separating their person from their disease. Physicians' commitment not to abandon their patients is of paramount importance.

Requests for assistance in dying only rarely evolve into fully considered requests for physician-assisted suicide or euthanasia. As illustrated in the case vignettes, a thorough exploration and understanding of the patient's experience and the reason the request is occurring at a given moment in time often yield avenues of "help" that are acceptable to almost all physicians and ethicists. These clinical summaries have been oversimplified to illustrate distinct levels of meaning. More often, multiple levels exist simultaneously, yielding several avenues for potential intervention. Rather than making any assumptions about what kind of help is being requested, the physician may ask the patient to help clarify by asking, "How were you hoping I could help?" Exploring a patient's request or wish does not imply an obligation to accede, but rather to seriously listen and to consider with an open mind. Even if the physician cannot directly respond to a rational request for a physician-assisted death because of personal, moral, or legal constraints, exploring, understanding, and expressing empathy can often be therapeutic.[30,31] In addition, the physician and the patient may be able to find some creative middle ground that is acceptable to both.[32,33] Finding common ground that can enhance the patient's comfort, dignity, and personal choice at death without compromising the physician's personal and professional values can be creative, challenging, and satisfying work for physicians.

### What Do Dying Persons Want Most from Their Physicians?

Most patients clearly do not want to die, but if they must, they would like to do so while maintaining their physical and personal integrity.[34] When faced with a patient expressing a wish for death, and a request for help, physicians (and others) should consider the following.

#### Listen and Learn from the Patient before Responding

Learning as much as possible about the patient's unique suffering and about exactly what is being requested is a vital first step. Physicians tend to be action-oriented, yet these problems only infrequently yield simple resolutions. This is not to say they are insoluble, but the patient is the initial guide to defining the problem and the range of acceptable interventions.

### Be Compassionate, Caring, and Creative

Comfort care is a far cry from "not doing anything." It is completely analogous to intensive medical care, only in this circumstance the care is directed toward the person and his or her suffering, not the disease. Dying patients need our commitment to creatively problem-solve and support them no matter where their illness may go. The rules and methods are not simple when applied to real persons, but the satisfaction and meaning of helping someone find his or her own path to a dignified death can be immeasurable.

### Promise to Be There until the End

Many people have personally witnessed or in some way encountered "bad deaths," though what this might mean to a specific patient is varied and unpredictable. Patients need our assurance that, if things get horrible, undignified, or intolerable, we will not abandon them, and we will continue to work with them to find acceptable solutions. Usually those solutions do not involve directly assisting death, but they may often involve the aggressive use of symptom-relieving measures that might indirectly hasten death.[3,35] We should be able to reassure all our patients that they will not die racked by physical pain, for it is now accepted practice to give increasing amounts of analgesic medicine until the pain is relieved even if it inadvertently shortens life. Many patients find this promise reassuring, for it both alleviates the fear of pain, and also makes concrete the physician's willingness to find creative, aggressive solutions.

### If Asked, Be Honest about Your Openness to the Possibility of Assisted Suicide

Patients who want to explore the physician's willingness to provide a potentially lethal prescription often fear being out of control, physically dependent, or mentally incapacitated, rather than simply fearing physical pain.[36] For many, the possibility of a controlled death if things become intolerable is often more important than the reality. Those who secretly hold lethal prescriptions or who have a physician who will entertain the possibility of such treatment feel a sense of control and possibility that, if things became intolerable, there will be a potential escape. Other patients will be adequately reassured to know that we can acknowledge the problem, talk about death, and actively search for acceptable alternatives, even if we cannot directly assist them.

### Try to Approach Intolerable End-of-Life Suffering with an Open Heart and an Open Mind

Though acceptable solutions can almost always be found through the aggressive application of comfort care principles, this is not a time for denial of the problem or for superficial solutions. If there are no good alternatives, what should the patient do? There is often a moment of truth for health care providers and families faced with a patient whom they care about who has no acceptable options. Physicians must not turn their backs, but continue to problem-solve, to be present, to help their patients find dignity in death.

### Do Not Forget Your Own Support

Working intensively with dying patients can be both enriching and draining. It forces us to face our own mortality, our abilities, and our limitations. It is vital to have a place where we can openly share our own grief, doubts, and uncertainties, as well as take joy in our small victories.[37] For us to deepen our understanding of the human condition and to help humanize the dying process for our patients and ourselves, we must learn to give voice to and share our own private experience of working closely with dying patients.

The patients with whom we engage at this level often become indelibly imprinted on our identities as professionals. Much like the death of a family member, the process that they go through and our willingness and ability to be there and to be helpful are often replayed and rethought. The intensity of these relationships and our ability to make a difference are often without parallel. Because the road is traveled by us all, but the map is poorly described, it is often an adventure with extraordinary richness and unclear boundaries.

## Notes

In memory of Arthur Schmale, MD, who taught me how to listen, learn, and take direction from the personal stories of dying patients.

1   Wanzer SH, Adelstein SJ, Cranford RE, et al. The physician's responsibility toward hopelessly ill patients. *N Engl J Med.* 1984;310:955–959.

2   Wanzer SH, Federman DO, Adelstein SJ, et al. The physician's responsibility toward hopelessly ill patients: a second look. *N Engl J Med.* 1989;320:844–849.

3   Council on Ethical and Judicial Affairs, American Medical Association. Decisions near the end of life. *JAMA.* 1992; 267:2229–2233.

4   Rhymes J. Hospice care in America. *JAMA.* 1990; 264:369–372.

5   Hastings Center Report. *Guidelines on the Termination of Life-Sustaining Treatment and the Care of the Dying.* New York: Hastings Center, 1987.

6   Zimmerman JM. *Hospice: Complete Care for the Terminally Ill.* Baltimore, MD: Urban & Schwarzenberg, 1981.

7   Quill T. *Death and Dignity: Making Choices and Taking Charge.* New York: W. W. Norton, 1993.

8   Aries P. *The Hour of Our Death.* New York: Vintage Books, 1982.

9   Kubler-Ross E. *On Death and Dying.* New York: Macmillan, 1969.

10  Richman J. A rational approach to rational suicide. *Suicide Life Threat Behav.* 1992; 22:130–141.

11  Foley KM. The treatment of cancer pain. *N Engl J Med.* 1989;313:84–95.

12  Kane RL, Bernstein L, Wales J, Rothenberg R. Hospice effectiveness in controlling pain. *JAMA.* 1985;253:2683–2686.

13  Twyeross RG, Lack SA. *Symptom Control in Far Advanced Cancer: Pain Relief.* London: Pitman Books, 1984.

14  Kerr IG, Some M, DeAngelis C, et al. Continuous narcotic infusion with patient-controlled analgesia for chronic cancer outpatients. *Ann Intern Med.* 1988;108:554–557.

15  Garfield C. *Psychosocial Care of the Dying Patient.* New York: McGraw-Hill International, 1978.

16  Conwell Y, Caine ED. Rational suicide and the right to die: reality and myth. *N Engl J Med.* 1991; 325:1100–1103.

17  Allenbeck P, Bolund C, Ringback G. Increased suicide rate in cancer patients. *J Clin Epidemiol.* 1989;42:611–616.

18  Breitbart W. Suicide in cancer patients. *Oncology.* 1989;49–55.

19  MacKenzie TB, Popkin MK. Suicide in the medical patient. *Int J Psychiatry Med.* 1987;17:3–22.

20  Cassel CK, Meier DE. Morals and moralism in the debates on euthanasia and assisted suicide. *N Engl J Med.* 1990;323:750–752.

21  Quill TE. Death and dignity: a case of individualized decision making. *N Engl J Med.* 1991;324:691–694.

22  Jecker NS. Giving death a hand: when the dying and the doctor stand in a special relationship. *J Am Geriatr Soc.* 1991;39:831–835.

23  Angell M. Euthanasia. *N Engl J Med.* 1988;319:1348–1350.

24  Brody H. Assisted death: a compassionate response to a medical failure. *N Engl J Med.* 1992; 327:1384–1388.

25 Quill TE, Cassel CK, Meier DE. Care of the hopelessly ill: potential clinical criteria for physician-assisted suicide. *N Engl J Med.* 1992;327:1380–1384.

26 Singer PA, Siegler M. Euthanasia: a critique. *N Engl J Med.* 1990;322:1881–1883.

27 Orentlicher D. Physician participation in assisted suicide. *JAMA.* 1989;262:1844–1845.

28 Gaylin WL, Kass R, Pellegrino ED, Siegler M. Doctors must not kill. *JAMA.* 1988;259:2139–2140.

29 Gomez CF. *Regulating Death: Euthanasia and the Case of the Netherlands.* New York: Free Press, 1991.

30 Novack DH. Therapeutic aspects of the clinical encounter. *J Gen Intern Med.* 1987;2:346–355.

31 Suchman AL, Matthews DA. What makes the doctor-patient relationship therapeutic: exploring the connexional dimension of medical care. *Ann Intern Med.* 1988;108:125–130.

32 Quill TE. Partnerships in patient care: a contractual approach. *Ann Intern Med.* 1983;98:228–234.

33 Fisher, R., Ury, W. *Getting to Yes: Negotiating Agreement Without Giving In.* Boston: Houghton Mifflin, 1981.

34 Cassel EJ. The nature of suffering and the goals of medicine. *N Engl J Med.* 1982;306:639–645.

35 Meier DE, Cassel CK. Euthanasia in old age: a case study and ethical analysis. *J Am Geriatr Soc.* 1983;31:294–298.

36 Van der Maas PJ, van Delden JJM, Pijnenborg L, Looman CWN. Euthanasia and other medical decisions concerning the end of life. *Lancet.* 1991;338:669–674.

37 Quill TE, Williams PR. Healthy approaches to physician stress. *Arch Intern Med.* 1990;150:1857–1861.

## The Chain of Safety
Charles R. Feldstein

"How do I die, Charles?" you whisper from the hospital bed.
"Do I just close my eyes?"

Your unanswered question
returns me to myself,
to a younger you,
to when my brothers and I
were small and walked down
by the wide stream
off Canterbury Road
after a hard rain
to watch branches, leaves
swept away
in the swirling water,
and you'd insist
that the four of us link hands,
as you held out yours
to start our Chain of Safety,
and we'd tread hand in hand
by the water's edge,
you in the lead.

But now I feel you leaving
the shoreline, Mom, and moving
by yourself into that place where
deep water and drowning are the same,
for the swirling water
has become safe and beautiful
to you, and I know
you will not reach out
to us even one more time,
yet how natural for me
to want you here, like
a hand that insists
on being held.

# Try to Remember Some Details
Yehuda Amichai

Try to remember some details. Remember the clothing
of the one you love
so that on the day of loss you'll be able to say: last seen
wearing such-and-such, brown jacket, white hat.
Try to remember some details. For they have no face
and their soul is hidden and their crying
is the same as their laughter,
and their silence and their shouting rise to one height
and their body temperature is between 98 and 104 degrees
and they have no life outside this narrow space
and they have no graven image, no likeness, no memory
and they have paper cups on the day of their rejoicing
and paper cups that are used once only.

Try to remember some details. For the world
is filled with people who were torn from their sleep
with no one to mend the tear,
and unlike wild beasts they live
each in his lonely hiding place and they die
together on battlefields
and in hospitals.

Yehuda Amichai, "Try to Remember Some Details," from *The Selected Poetry of Yehuda Amichai*, trans. Chana Bloch and Stephan Mitchell. © 1986 by Yehuda Amichai. Reprinted by permission of HarperCollins Publishers, Inc.

# Index to Authors

# About the Editors

Larry R. Churchill, PhD, holds the Ann Geddes Stahlman Chair in Medical Ethics, Department of Medicine, Center for Clinical and Research Ethics, Vanderbilt University. He also holds appointments in Vanderbilt's Divinity School and in the Department of Philosophy. From 1988 to 1998 he was chair of the Department of Social Medicine, University of North Carolina at Chapel Hill School of Medicine. His recent research is focused on justice and U.S. health policy, the ethics of research with human subjects, and the relationship between bioethics and ordinary moral experience.

Sue E. Estroff, PhD, is a professor in the Department of Social Medicine and an adjunct professor in the Departments of Anthropology and Psychiatry, School of Medicine and College of Arts and Sciences, University of North Carolina at Chapel Hill. She is the author of numerous cultural analyses of schizophrenia and other severe persistent psychiatric disorders, focusing most recently on the topics of contested identity and conflicting representations between medical and psychiatric formulations and those of people with schizophrenia. Her other current work includes cultural analysis of consent in the context of experimental fetal surgery, exploring moral quandaries in the production of knowledge, and examining the roles of social and cultural factors in violence in the lives of people with schizophrenia.

Gail E. Henderson, PhD, is a professor in the Department of Social Medicine, School of Medicine, and an adjunct professor in the Department of Sociology, College of Arts and Sciences, University of North Carolina at Chapel Hill. Her teaching and research interests include health and inequality, heath and health care in China, and research ethics. She has extensive experience with qualitative and quantitative data collection and analysis, as well as with conceptual and empirical cross-disciplinary research and analysis. In China, she has taught social science research methods to clinical epidemiologists, and conducted research ethics training workshops for HIV/AIDS researchers. Her current research focuses on ethical issues in gene transfer clinical trials and cancer genetic epidemiology studies, and understanding how research ethics committees in China and Africa oversee international collaborative research.

Nancy M. P. King, JD, is a professor in the Department of Social Medicine, University of North Carolina at Chapel Hill School of Medicine. Her scholarly interests focus on individual and policy-level decision making in health care and research, and the relationship between bioethics and law. She teaches and advises on human subjects research ethics and health care ethics locally, nationally, and internationally, addressing issues ranging from literature and medicine to end-of-life court decisions to genetic databases. Her current research and most recent publications address informed consent in gene transfer research.

Jonathan Oberlander, PhD, is an associate professor in the Department of Social Medicine at the University of North Carolina at Chapel Hill, where he teaches health policy in the School of Medicine and Department of Political Science. He is a Greenwall Foundation Faculty Scholar in Bioethics and the author of *The Political Life of Medicare* (University of Chicago Press). His research and teaching interests include health politics and policy, Medicare, health care reform, and medical care rationing. Current research focuses on market-based strategies for Medicare reform, the politics of incremental and state-led health reform, and a study of the Oregon Health Plan.

Ronald P. Strauss, DMD, PhD, is a professor in the Department of Social Medicine, School of Medicine, and Dental Friends Distinguished Professor and Chair, Department of Dental Ecology, School of Dentistry, University of North Carolina at Chapel Hill. He is both a sociologist of medicine and a dentist, with a research focus on stigmatization and the social impacts of chronic health problems including craniofacial anomalies and HIV/AIDS. He is the director of the Social and Behavioral Sciences Research Core of the UNC Center for AIDS Research. Current research includes an oral health disparities research project in Hawaii, a study of health promotion in low-income workplaces in eastern North Carolina, a study that examines stigma experience related to TB and HIV in south Thailand, and a multisite project that evaluates quality of life in adolescents with facial differences.

Library of Congress Cataloging-in-Publication Data
The social medicine reader.—2nd ed.
p. ; cm.
Includes bibliographical references and index.
ISBN 0-8223-3555-7 (v. 1 : cloth : alk. paper)
ISBN 0-8223-3568-9 (v. 1 : pbk. : alk. paper)
ISBN 0-8223-3580-8 (v. 2 : cloth : alk. paper)
ISBN 0-8223-3593-X (v. 2 : pbk. : alk. paper)
ISBN 0-8223-3556-5 (v. 3 : cloth : alk. paper)
ISBN 0-8223-3569-7 (v. 3 : pbk. : alk. paper)
1. Social medicine.
[DNLM: 1. Social Medicine—Collected Works.
2. Ethics, Clinical—Collected Works. 3. Health
Policy—Collected Works. 4. Professional-Patient
Relations—Collected Works. 5. Sick Role—Col-
lected Works. 6. Socioeconomic Factors—Collected
Works. 7. Terminal Care—Collected Works.
WA 31 S67803 2005] I. King, Nancy M. P.
RA418.S6424 2005    362.1'042—dc22    2005010301